# AYURVEDA FOREVER WELLBEING

*A Treasury of Holistic Recommendations*



Meta B. Doherty

MOTILAL BANARSIDASS
SINCE 1903 IN INDOLOGY

MOTILAL BANARSIDASS PUBLISHERS
PRIVATE LIMITED • DELHI

*First Indian Edition: Delhi, 2017*

Published in arrangement with
LOTUS PRESS
P.O. Box 325, Twin Lakes, WI 53181 USA
lotuspress@lotuspress.com, www.lotuspress.com



ISBN: 978-81-208-4096-6

*Also available at*

MOTILAL BANARSIDASS
41 U.A. Bungalow Road, Jawahar Nagar, Delhi 110 007
8 Mahalaxmi Chamber, 22 Bhulabhai Desai Road, Mumbai 400 026
203 Royapettah High Road, Mylapore, Chennai 600 004
236, 9th Main III Block, Jayanagar, Bengaluru 560 011
8 Camac Street, Kolkata 700 017
Ashok Rajpath, Patna 800 004
Chowk, Varanasi 221 001

DISCLAIMER
This book is not intended to treat, diagnose or prescribe. The information contained herein is in no way to be considered as a substitute for a consultation with a duly licensed health care professional.

FOR SALE IN SOUTH ASIA ONLY

Library of Congress Number 2013933189

*Published by*
Motilal Banarsidass Publishers Private Limited
*www.mlbd.com* • *mlbd@mlbd.com*
*Printed by* Gopsons Papers Ltd

# Salutations to the Energy of New Beginnings Sri:

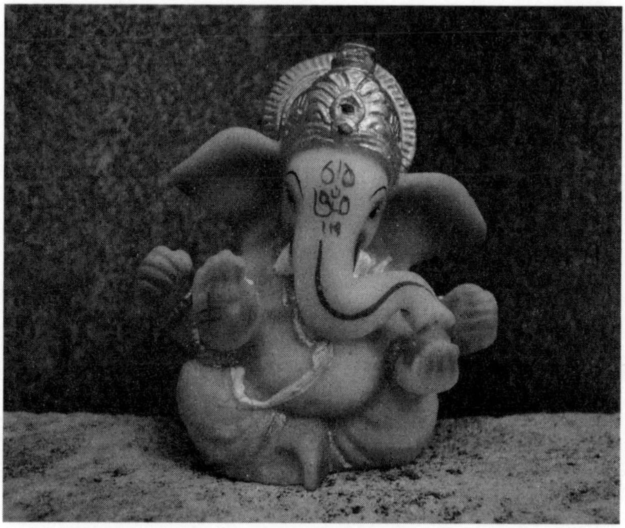

*Elephants are still used to remove obstacles in remote areas. When an elephant is young, one leg is tied to a post to prevent it from wandering. As an adult, it can easily uproot the post yet its past experience prevents it from trying.*

*May our obstacles be removed.*

*May this endeavor be victorious.*
**Jaya Ganesha!**

## Dedicated to all who offer healing and to all who receive healing, with gratitude to

**Dr Rajen Cooppan** for the foundation of all my learning.

**Dr Subhash** and **Dr Visakh** for their discussion of Keraleeya Ayurveda. To experience how love heals, visit them for treatments.

**Simon Borg-Olivier** for elucidating the why of yoga in terms of human anatomy, physiology and consciousness.

**Mark Whitwell** for linking me to the Yoga of Krishnamacharya; and for linking to all people as friends.

**Bhagyashree Sawrikar** (Bachelor Ayurvedic Medical Science, India) for the information on Mother and Child Health.

**Sejal Shah** (Bachelor Ayurvedic Medical Science, India) for her suggestions and reviewing all the information in this book.

**My friends in Sneha Ayus Sangha**, our ayurvedic social and study group in Perth.

**Gabriel Zahra** at Upper Crust Cooking School, Perth, for opening the door to ayurveda and Sattwa Café cookbook.

**Dr David Frawley** and **Shankar.**

**Dr John Douillard** and **Sita.**

**Geoff** for the Photoshopping.

**My family and friends** world-wide.

**Santosh** and **Lotus Press** for its substantial contribution to the wellbeing of people through the publication of ayurvedic material. And om shanti **Shanta**.

# Contents

## PART THREE: Embellish the Recommendations 107



## PART FOUR: Suggested Reading and Reference 152

# INTRODUCTION

Ayurveda is the Science of Life that originated in the distant past (over 40,000 years ago) on the Indian mainland. The principles of Ayurveda are rooted in the intense and astute study of the laws of nature and how they apply to human life.

The principles, when understood, can be used effectively to shape a life filled with wellness and health.

The need of the hour in modern society all across the globe, is a simple yet effective medical science that places the power of choice back into the hands of the average person.

Ayurveda is that Science, and Meta's second book on some of the principles of Ayurveda, is a welcome addition to the books currently available on Ayurvedic principles, that can serve the modern person today.

It is uncomplicated yet holds true to the sublime principles of life. This book will become a handbook to many who seek better health and a more fulfilled life.

**Dr Rajen Cooppan (MBChB, MD, Dip Ayu)**
**Course Developer and Facilitator for**
**The Foundation Training in Clinical Ayurveda**

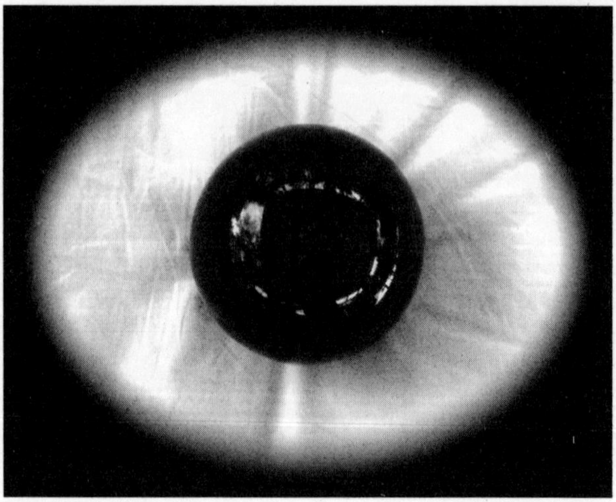

# PRACTICAL TRUTHS ABOUT AYURVEDA

The ancient scriptures of Ayurveda – samhitas – are written in the holy language, Sanskrit. Sanskrit was the primary liturgical language of Hinduism, Jainism and Buddhism. When Buddhism became popularised in Kerala, South India, Ayurveda along with Sanskrit might have set foot. But the differences in the medicines used and the treatment methods reveal one thing – even before the advent of Ayurveda, there were many ongoing unique traditional treatment modalities. So it should be believed that these traditional practices of herbal medicines helped the development of Ayurveda here.

The unique use of certain herbs, special treatment procedures, vast pharmacological knowledge together with the ability to successfully treat and cure diseases like small pox, well-developed toxicology and the speciality of marma chikitsa (pressure points) by the traditional practitioners in Kerala show their extensive knowledge in this stream of medicine.

Kerala's rich Ayurvedic tradition is believed to be passed on from the great seer Parashurama to Ashta vaidyas. The Parashurama was considered to be an incarnation of Lord Vishnu, preserver and sustainer of the universe. Ayurveda will be the hand of the lord for maintaining health and wellbeing of the universe.

**Dr P. S. Subhash & Dr P. S.Visakh (Son of Dr Subhash)**

AYUR DARA

|| loka : samastha : sukhino bavanthu ||

"In all realities, for all beings, may there be the blessings of ease of heartspace"

**Vypeen Island-Kochi - Kerala, India**

# Practical Truths About Yoga

Ayurveda takes care of ayus, embodied life: soul, mind, senses and body in intelligent communication. It is often said that hatha yoga is the sister science of ayurveda. Hatha means literally 'force' and so hatha yoga is the physical yoga that deals with the forces we manifest and harness within our body.

According to the contemporary physical Yoga Master Yang Zhen Hua there are only three things you need to do to realise yoga in your body:

1. Unblock the blockages of the natural energy within
2. Circulate the energy (prana) through the subtle channels (nadis) of the body
3. Just sit back and enjoy the natural state of paradise

1. To 'unblock the blockages of energy' in the body the most important aspects are to be relaxed and natural in movement and posture. Physical yoga focuses on 12 key relaxation points or bridges within the body that are all under both conscious and unconscious control. One of these places is the diaphragm. Hence, the ability to first restore natural breathing and later learn to control the breath is paramount to good yoga. Natural movements are those that do not involve any sense of stretching or tensing muscles. So even though regular practice of physical yoga makes you very flexible and strong because it does lengthen muscles and activate various muscles groups, the natural movements of yoga should not feel like stretching or tensing anything. To work like this of course needs regular non-aggressive practice that is honest and truthful without the ego dominating or it being goal-oriented. In other words we are not trying to do perfect postures but trying to feel good in a natural way.

2. In order to circulate energy within the channels (nadis) of the body (which include blood vessels) the 7 circulatory pumps are developed and used to their maximum. Of these circulatory pumps the heart is the least effective and so its use is discouraged until the effects of all other pumps are maximised. The other six circulatory pumps harness the forces associated with gravity, muscle activity, respiration, posture, muscle co-activation, and movement. In order to get the oxygen carried in the blood into the actual cells of the body, breath-control is essential. Natural diaphragmatic breathing and eventually the controlled hypoventilation (reduced

breathing) involved with real yogic breath-control (pranayama) causes an increase in levels of carbon dioxide in the blood that dilates blood vessels and hence brings more blood to essential organs. Increased carbon dioxide is also essential for the exchange of gases at a cellular level to get the oxygen into the cells via the Bohr effect.

3. Once the blockages caused by tension and incorrect posture and movement are eliminated and yogic techniques have been used to move energy (prana), the body experiences union and uniform communication within. Energy flow and internal healing occur on all levels. This connection and internal communication can be experienced as energy, mental clarity and emotional bliss. The yogic teaching however is not to wait for this state to arrive but rather to lovingly (isvara pranidhana) make your best attempt to reach it (tapas), yet without aggression or violence in body or mind to yourself or others (ahimsa), and when all is said and done, to then be content (santosa) with the outcome.

As in ayurveda, the internal benefits of yoga are of partial use unless they manifest externally. So the idea in yoga is that the practitioner practices to improve self-love, passion, making their best attempt at all things, being non-violent and developing the ability to be content or happy with their place in life. Ideally it is these ideas that yoga practice can spread and foster. The communication nurtured within us in hatha yoga that can give us healing, health and internal communication can then be a model for us all to give healing, health and loving union to our families, friends, the earth itself and all who live on it.

**Simon Borg-Olivier, MSc, BAppSc (Physiotherapy), MAPA.**

**yoga**synergy

Yoga Synergy, Sydney, Australia

# Practical Truths About Ayurveda and Yoga

Meta Doherty and the ancient world give us a profound gift. You hold it in your hands. The principles of health and healing from the ancient wisdom perspective of Ayurveda is her understanding and life's work. Ayurveda reveals to us that Reality, that which beats our heart, moves our breath and all relatedness is none other than a nurturing force, continuity and certainty. It is utterly on you, in you, as you and all your relationships. Yoga, a subset of Ayurveda is your ease full participation in the given Reality, the wonder, extreme intelligence and extreme functioning that is your life.

**Thank you Meta.**

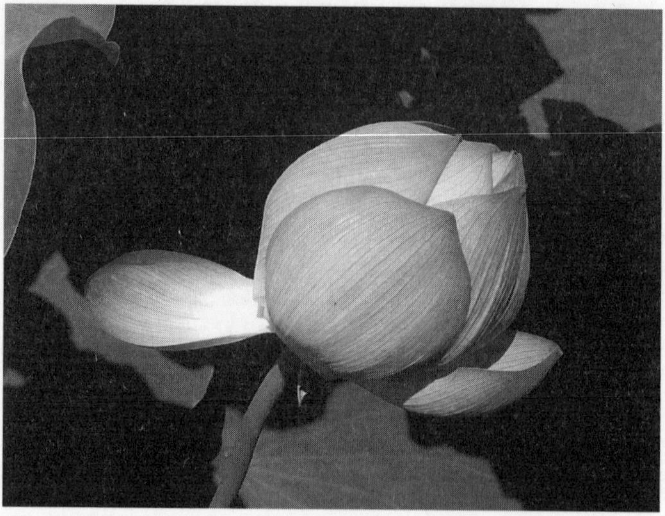

**Mark Whitwell, author** *Yoga of Heart* **and** *The Promise*

# Part One

## The First Year

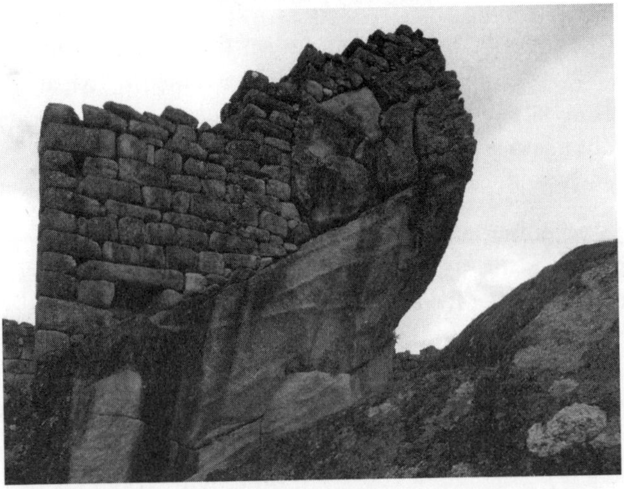

THE COMMON SENSE REMEDIES OF AYURVEDA do not work fast, although you may notice some immediate results. They work over a longer term. The recommendations become lifestyle changes and work deeply, restoring the tissues and functions of the body. If we follow one suggestion for one week and expect a result, we will consider ayurveda ineffective. Ayurveda is the knowledge that promotes life, holistic health and longevity.

To join 'CLUB AYURVEDA' we need to actually follow the suggestions. Everything is to be found in the experience, not reading or talking about it or what it can do for us. You never know. Resistance to the doing of these suggestions and to routines in general is created by the agitated state of our minds and sustained by our overactive culture. This state of mind holds old habits in place. We claim that routine robs us of spontaneity but a haphazard life is not an exciting life, it is mindlessness in action, our own minds running a pre-programmed show. Ayurveda and yoga address this level, the mind, for it is here that the changes begin. We move forward mentally and instil new habits alongside old ones. Eventually the old habits become the road no longer taken.

The strategies of ayurveda are all directed at revealing our innate wisdom that has been overshadowed by actions and beliefs that are probably not conducive to wellbeing and positive evolution. Ayurveda is about taking care of the body, the senses and the mind and the coordination of those aspects by our directional intelligence, spirit. Every lineage of ayurveda has connection to the original teachings, followed precisely or perhaps modified through subjectivity, experience, climate and available herbs. It is marvellous how much information is available yet the volume can be overwhelming. The approach that follows is simple and one of many. Please allow that all, some or even none of what follows will work for you.

Think of these words as a guided tour on the big bus of life: "Ladies and gentlemen, if you look to your right you will see…" Meanwhile, you're looking left! That's real too. Our own mindful primary experience is what matters. When you go to the restroom during the tour you have not missed out on your own life.

Introduce one practice every two weeks. If you like it, stick with it. If it takes longer, fine, there is no rush. Ask yourself where the resistance lies. Remember that above all we are working with the mind and need it onside. It is possible to skip any recommendation the week it is presented. Or return when the changes already established make it more agreeable. Or let it go. Really, only one well-entrained recommendation will open the way for others to follow. Working with a friend in this will be of great support as you progress together and amuse each other with your experiences.

Nothing new under the sun? Your interaction with these ancient teachings creates a new event.

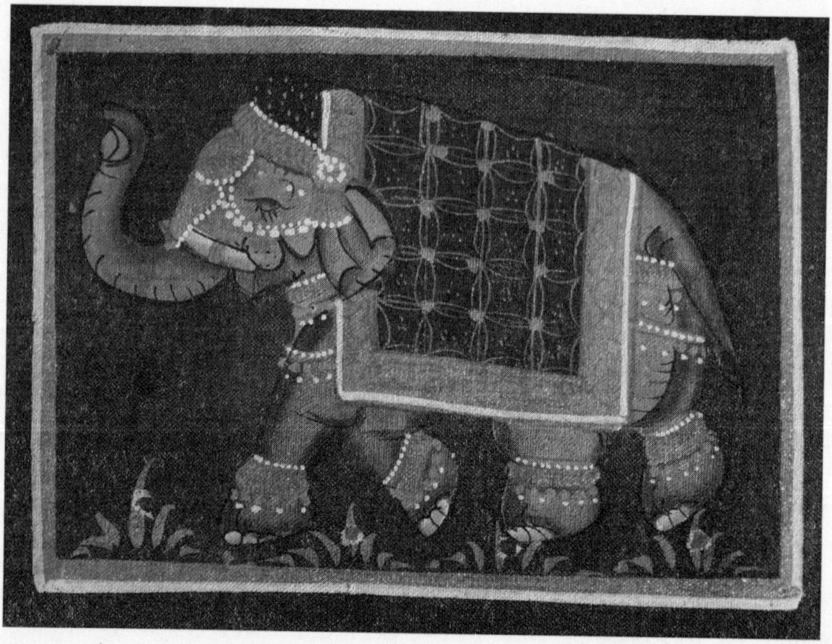

# Weeks 1 & 2
## CARE of the MOUTH and SENSE of TASTE

### GOOD MORNING!

Each morning, every morning, include these procedures in any order before taking anything by mouth:

1. Brush your teeth with a non-foaming herbal tooth preparation. Some brands include Weleda Plant Gel, Vicco Vajradanti Tooth Powder and Monkey Brand Charcoal Tooth Powder. We are encouraging our oral secretions to be thin rather than sticky.

2. Clean the entire surface of your tongue well with a tongue cleaner or small spoon, like shaving your tongue. Relax so that the implement can remove the impurities from the back without harm, moving further back day by day.

3. Perform gandush by mixing a *small* amount of salt and turmeric powder into warm water and use as a mouthwash and a gargle. Rinse with water.

Even better instead, perform gandush (if you find it comfortable) by swishing 1-teaspoon cold-pressed sesame oil in the mouth for 5 minutes. This is highly effective in cleansing the lymphatic system. Spit the oil out in a suitable place and rinse with water.

Rinse well with water after eating and floss once a day or as suggested by your dentist. All of these recommendations are most effective first thing in the morning. Before bed, clean your teeth as usual.

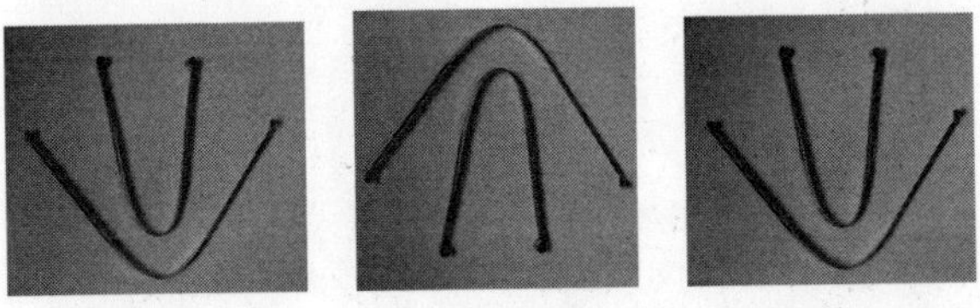

Options: Add 1 drop of tea tree or thyme oil to either mouthwash as a disinfectant. (Do not swallow.)

For sore throat mix two teaspoons turmeric in two teaspoons unfired honey and ingest ½-teaspoon six times per day until symptoms subside.

Now it's up to you to take these words on the page, this idea in your mind, and translate it into action.

This may be the second most confrontational recommendation so good luck!

## Weeks 3 & 4 — HOT WATER

Bring to boil good quality water that has not been previously boiled. If using tap water leave the pot uncovered to release waste gases. Sip as warm as possible and give your attention to the experience. If the water is too heating, let it cool more. The outcome of any of these recommendations is non-conditional. That means that we cannot be guaranteed of a prescribed effect because Nature is working with each of us as an individual.

Hot water is such a potent detoxifier, in part due to its reduced surface tension, that if you drink too much you will feel ill. That is an indication that the liver cannot detoxify the impurities at the rate it is receiving them.

Many people have warm water first thing in the morning with lemon juice. Lemon is a good support for the liver. Yet beginning the day with plain hot water is ideal because it is in its purest form. Make sure you've completed your oral hygiene first.

Increase the amount of hot water slowly up to three cups a day. In that way consumption of tea, even herbal tea and coffee will decrease. You need not drink a full cup at a time. Some people find that hot water with a sprinkle of ginger powder with meals helps their digestion. Some people find that ginger powder tea makes them too hot or causes insomnia. Some people find that drinking with meals fills them up too fast. As with every suggestion, experiment with where and how it works best for you. Take things slowly, as that is how we make lasting changes.

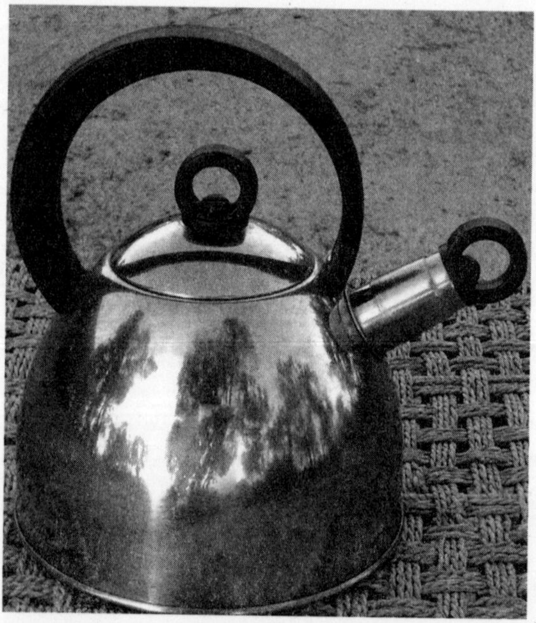

# Weeks 5 & 6 — AMA-REDUCING BROTH

Ama is the rubbish that accrues in our bodies and minds from incomplete digestion. Chewing over the same stressful thoughts is mental indigestion.

We add the following alkaline broth to our diet each day during this time.

- 1 carrot cut into small pieces
- 2 stalks of celery cut into small pieces
- a small amount of chopped spinach
- 1 potato cut into small pieces
- 500 ml quality water
- dash of asafoetida (hing) available in Indian grocery stores
- pinch of dried tarragon or handful of fresh
- ½-tablespoon Braggs Liquid Aminos to taste or ½-teaspoon salt
- 1-teaspoon ghee (clarified butter) or oil of your choice
- 2 generous cups (500 ml) quality water

1. Combine the vegetables and water and bring to boil in a soup pot. Cover and simmer 20 minutes.
2. Add the remaining ingredients and cook 5 minutes more. Begin to cool.
3. Strain the vegetables for a clear broth, blend for a thick soup or eat as is. The ideal is to drink the broth only, perhaps from a small bowl.

Makes two large serves. Please do not make up a large amount and freeze. Ayurveda categorically recommends eating foods cooked fresh each day using fresh ingredients. If meals are replaced with this, weight loss will occur but don't make a mono-diet of it.

Each person will make this his/her own way. One friend simmers it uncovered for more than 20 minutes until the flavor of the broth condenses and the vegetables are just fiber to be composted. Another cannot think of discarding the vegetables so cooks it just the 20 and adds the spinach in the last five. In that way it's a soup. How would you like to prepare it? This broth can be considered part of lunch and dinner, or morning and afternoon tea.

Re-warm it on the stove top before serving. Adding split mung beans, about 1 tablespoon, is a variation and will enhance nutrition. Soak them first and begin cooking just the beans for 10 minutes, skimming the top before adding the vegetables. After these two weeks, cook as often as you like, ideally once a week.

# Weeks 7 & 8 — YOGA

Ayurveda recognises a range of physical movement, the robust type such as sport, jogging, swimming, hiking, etc. where the heart rate is elevated and the muscles, circulation and sweating functions are stimulated, and energy enhancing movements such as tai chi, chi kung and yoga. In the latter the breathing lengthens rather than shortens and one feels they could move at that pace all day. The heart rate is not elevated yet the muscles, circulation and sweating functions are activated.

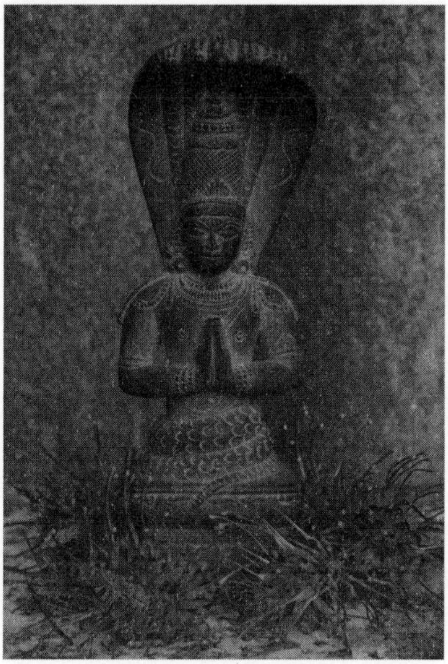

The Sage Patanjali

Yoga helps stretch and strengthen muscles; alternately expands and compresses organs of the abdomen, thus preventing stagnation of digestion and elimination; releases endorphins and so relaxes your mind and thence body; deepens and slows your breathing and so relaxes your emotional mind and helps you breathe less overall; and fosters balance, integration and experience of altogether essential unity. Traditional yoga also includes chanting and discussion of ideas as found in yoga texts.

Your practice of yoga or any ayurvedic recommendation should not cause disruption to anyone, including yourself and those with whom you live. To plonk yourself down in the middle of the living room and announce you are practicing yoga at the busiest time of day is asking to be stepped on in more ways than one.

Please read *BEFORE* beginning and refer back to substantiate your experience with these guidelines.

- Use these programs at home and when you travel. Program A is the entry. Become comfortable with it, especially your breathing and ease. It is okay to refer to the autoshape figures and instructions in the early stages as often as necessary. The more attention given, the sooner you will be free of that interruption.

- A balanced practice will be a plait of moving dynamically, staying in poses and resting. All breathing is through the nostrils. If you breathe through your mouth, begin to transfer comfort to nostril breathing. Adjust each posture so that you can do that easily.

- If in doubt as to a posture's suitability, check in with yourself and your health care provider.

- During your menstrual period focus on rest, soft breathing and contemplation. Pause your postures at this time.

- During early pregnancy do not strongly twist, fold or stretch the abdomen. See Part Three MOTHER and CHILD HEALTH for some safe beginners' postures. During the 2$^{nd}$ and 3$^{rd}$ trimesters let your body and intuition be your guides. I have read authors say do and don't practice at this time. I practiced yoga including inversions until the beginning of the 9$^{th}$ month when I started getting contractions so I stopped the inversions. What experience are you conveying to yourself and your child with your actions? After the birth of your baby, rest is more important than exercise. Let yourself grow slowly back into your yoga practice.

- Towards menopause include more time in the meditative state as the hormonal system is influenced by the state of the mind. With menopause include all postures, even in gentler form, so as to keep body systems functioning.

- Wait 2 hours after eating, more or less, to begin. Work on a firm yet comfortable surface. Do not practice in a draft.

- This format is changeable which reflects our current state of being. We can always move out of a posture sooner or stay in a posture longer by letting our breathing rate indicate our ease. We can practice dynamically and not stay in any pose. We can rest more or less between postures.

- Our enjoyment helps us remain with inner awareness regardless of outer circumstances. That means that even as the world continues to happen outwardly, we do our own thing. Practicing yoga as presented in these programs is when body, breath and mind are integrated as your experience; you feel and are attentive to what you are doing. This state is not limited to the yoga mat.

- Keep your spine long through your crown (your anterior fontanel) and legs before you bend or twist it. Adjust the effort to the movement. Anything more is strain, anything less is lax. If you wish to alter a posture to greater comfort, do. Yoga fosters reflection and there is no such thing as yoga police. ("We've come on a call that you are not doing certified textbook yoga.")

- The sympathetic nervous system will contract all muscles in sympathy if one part of the body is being challenged beyond its current capacity. We can override that and keep some parts strong for safety and some parts relaxed. In all the weeks that follow, our face and throat are relaxed with an inner smile.

- The parasympathetic nervous system restores, among other organ-specific actions, a slower heart and breath rate after sympathetic activation. It threads through active practice and supine rest.

- Enteric nerves throughout the digestive system spark food processing and gut feelings independent of the brain. Besides the pause in eating, our practice is more effective when we feel safe.

- It is advisable to have an instructor observe your practice periodically in case the instructions have been misleading.

- If you wish, acknowledge commencement and completion with a chosen gesture, thought, prayer and/or affirmation ritual.

- Make sure you are fully grounded afterwards, that is, you remember the rules of the road before driving!

- Make ready an area, choosing a time that will be available most days. Once the momentum is going, it will be easy staying up on the yoga wave. Your practice will open itself before you. And the ride? To infinity and beyond! and deeper and broader into what life offers.

Lie down now and test the five postures to get the flow before reading about them. Look at the autoshape figures and do them even if you hold the book in your hand.

## PROGRAM A

Practice Program A and move, breathe and rest with it three to seven times a week. These postures are all done supported by the earth so that we can create an internal tapestry of structure woven with comfort. They are considered a quiet practice, suitable even before sleep.

Blessings on your experience of yoga.

### SEMI SUPINE

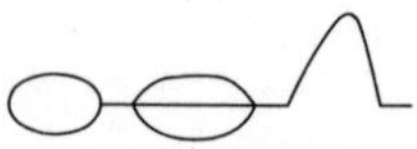

This horizontal supported pose allows for relaxing, centering and commencing awareness of the breath. If this is all that is done after hours of standing and sitting it will rehydrate our intervertebral discs, giving renewal to our spines for the rest of the day. For that purpose, 12 minutes rest is suggested.

Start with normal breathing through the nose, abdomen soft, expanding slightly and subsiding slightly for 6 breaths. Continue into the postures with breathing awareness when you are ready. We may take longer breaths and slower breaths without them being loud or hardening the body. If you find the breath is getting out of synch with the postures, start again from point of choice. If you find the mind is a short or long distance from your body and breathing, draw it close. Engage these postures and suggestions with a spirit of inquiry as to your affinity with them.

### APANASANA

"energy of elimination pose"

*exhale* ⟶

⟵ *inhale*

Apana is the energy of the lower body responsible for all downward movements. It can get unbalanced as we hold on, wanting things to stay the same forever. We can also do this pose one knee at a time with the other leg in semi-supine. Although the outward movement is simple, the inner one massages the organs with the breath and the help of gravity. Begin exhaling, move into the pose. Begin inhaling, move out. Do this dynamically with the breath four times and then stay in the more tucked aspect for 4 breaths. Then return the legs to semi supine.

## JATHARA PARIVRITTI

"revolved stomach movement"

legs move, hips roll

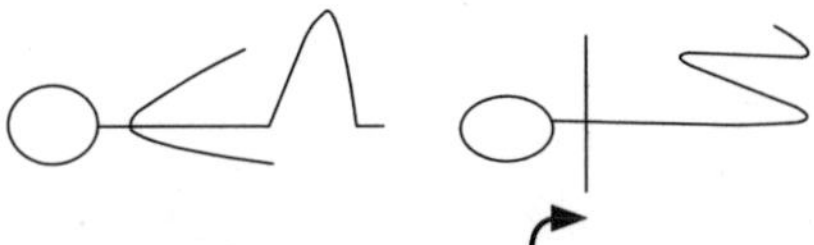

*inhale* *exhale*

This twist comfortably rotates the spine and abdomen. Begin with body and legs centered in semi supine, arms slightly away from the torso. Start the exhale and then lower your knees to the right; start the inhale and effortlessly move your legs to semi supine. Commence the exhalation, then lower legs to the left and commence the inhalation before moving easily back to center. Do this dynamically with the breath leading the movement for four pairs, then exhale and stay to the right for 4 breaths. Keep your shoulder blades wide and relaxed outward from your spine with your arms making room for your legs. Inhale, return to center; exhale, legs move to the left and stay for 4 breaths, body woven with comfort and form. Inhale to semi supine.

## DWI PADA PITHAM

"two legged table"

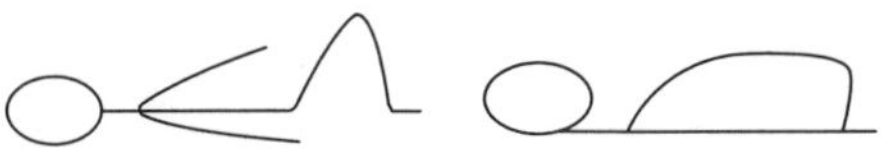

*inhale* ⟶

⟵ *exhale*

This is a back arch and partial inversion. After the initial exhale, lift your hips vertebra-by-vertebra starting from the tailbone on the inhalations, as many as you wish, and lower vertebra by vertebra on the exhalations from the neck, as many as you need to be present to the sensations. If you stay in the pose take some of the weight off your spine by pressing down through your arms where they join your torso and keeping your hips buoyant, thighs and feet even. Allow the back of your neck to lengthen but not completely flatten. How comfortable are you in your steadiness? If you are not, you are straining. If you are too relaxed the pose will seem harder to maintain. As your breath lengthens you could start the inhale and roll up on one inhalation, arms moving overhead, and start the exhale before rolling down on one exhalation, arms lowering to your sides. Do this dynamically four times, and then stay up in the pose for 4 breaths. Exhale down. Whatever your experience with these movements and breathing, that is yoga.

## SUPINE

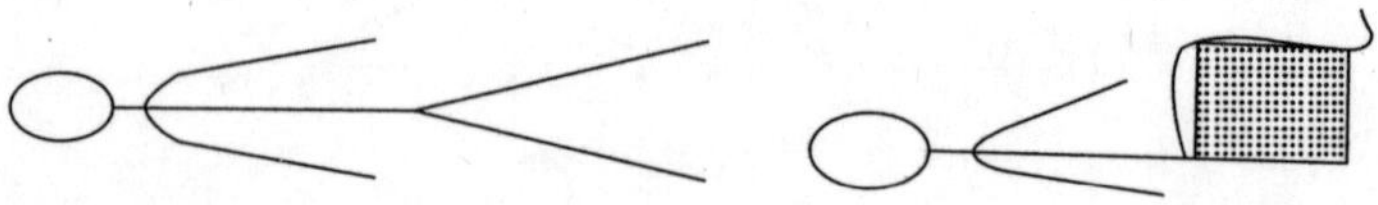

It is also possible to put a bolster under the backs of your thigh-knee area so that your legs can be extended and your lower back relaxed. Put a small folded towel under your head if needed. Rest with natural breathing, relaxed diaphragm, for 5 minutes staying present in your experience. Feel your body on solid ground. Feel yourself relax from the inside out.

## Weeks 9 & 10 — ABHYANGA

To help mobilize the ama in our tissues, relax our nervous system and silken our skin, we perform a self-massage every 2-3 days. Ideal times are first thing in the morning before your shower (make sure the space is warm) or in the late afternoon. Another good time is before bed. For many people the time of choice centers around shower time.

1. Warm about 7 teaspoons of cured sesame oil or other oil (see below) to just over body temperature. Adjust this amount to your body's surface area and absorption.
2. Working from your face down, apply oil with an open hand in long strokes on straight areas and circular movements over joints, clockwise on abdomen and going down to your feet. There may be some areas you cannot reach.
3. Do this massage focused on yourself so you can develop self-referral, a feedback mechanism based on intuition. What feels good is what is right, so your massage can be gentle, creative, brisk, etc.
4. Leave oil on for about 20 minutes, dressed in an old sweatshirt, pants and socks that you will donate to the cause. They will never be the same again. Do not rev up or go outside, but rather rest and stay warm. Oil and warmth open the body's channels to assist cleansing. You may find that you begin sweating which is a sign that your self-spa is working. You could stay in the moment, chanting, breathing or a further massage of face, hands, feet and ears during this time. I like to lie down under a blanket in semi-supine and lengthen my breathing. Do you find that you cannot pause for 20 minutes? That you feel a force trying to move you on? It's the mind. Think of something else for a few seconds and the urge will dissipate. If you find yourself getting chilled proceed to the next step.
5. Shower or bathe in warm water to remove the oil. Soap is not recommended for everyone, as it can be drying and caustic, especially to the genital area. A minimal amount of oil left in your pores is acceptable. As an alternative to soap combine chickpea flour with water or milk to create a "batter" and use this on your skin in the shower. Like soap, it may be too drying for you.

## WHICH OIL TO USE

If you are feeling cool or cold and your skin is dry use SESAME OIL. If you are feeling hot and the weather is hot, use COCONUT OIL. If you run hot and the weather is cool, use sunflower oil. If you are feeling cool, lethargic and heavy use MUSTARD and SESAME OIL 50/50. Only the sesame oil is cured. Adjust the temperature of the oil you use to your pleasure, warming just slightly or warming more. If you find after the twenty minutes there is a lot of oil just sitting on your skin, use less. If this is the case for your whole body perform abhyanga only once a week. If you practice dry brushing to feel stimulated (or the like), still use some oil to prevent harming the skin due to friction. Use cold-pressed oils, organic is best.

If you have skin, circulatory or immune imbalance, self-massage may be contraindicated. Otherwise, an easy start is with a face, ear, hand or foot massage. Try massaging your hands or ears now, even without oil.

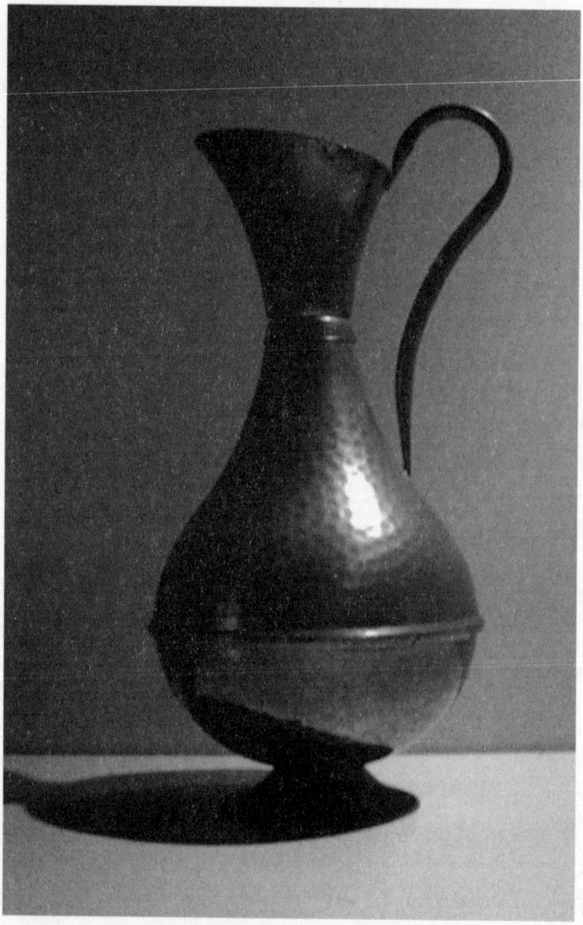

## CURING SESAME OIL

1. Pour the contents of one bottle of cold-pressed sesame oil (not Chinese sesame oil) into a small saucepan and add 2 mini-drops of water.
2. With complete attention, heat the oil and water until the water drops reach 212 degrees F = 100 degrees C and rise to the top spluttering. This happens rather quickly. Any more heat at this point could render the oil unusable and could eventually ignite the oil. Chain yourself to the stove if you have a tendency to wander. Option: look into the pan and watch the oil swirl.
3. Turn off the heat immediately.
4. When the oil cools, return it to the dark glass bottle.
5. Warm the required amount from this stock for your massage, maybe in a small glass bottle in some hot water. This oil is now appropriate for gandush too. There is no orifice into which sesame oil cannot be introduced.

# Weeks 11 & 12 — MEDITATION

This word has many associations so perhaps it would be better to begin with analogy.

Imagine if all you ever experienced was to go and do and be in the world outwardly and you had no place to return to, no place you could rest. Meditation is the return home. It opens the space of having a life without having to act or create strategies or have opinions. It is like the exhale part of the breath. It gentles our minds like a soft rain and like any fluid immersion, changes the energetic field around us.

Thinking is what the mind does and meditation does start with thinking; it can also experience a quieter, more focused state. Thoughts decrease and peace and stillness of a calmer mind prevail. From this state arises more clarity. It can be used to investigate objects and concepts on a deeper and more accurate basis. It can be used to receive insight from those objects. It can watch thoughts move through, it can enjoy non-analysis. It can allow some dismantling of ideas set in stone and know its spacious nature. It can laugh at its own antics and not take things so seriously.

There are many strategies to enable the mind to be present in its "best possible form" and the ideal one is that which is easy and agreeable to you. The mind assumes the shape of what we are thinking, so choose a thought or image that will benefit you. In reading this, you may already have a meditative practice. If not, consider as an example, some people would like to have a deeper connection to our sun and its characteristics of warmth, brilliance and energy. They could research facts about it, keep more in touch with it throughout the day, feel its warmth, imagine its energy (the mind boggles) and then when sitting formally could "be with their sun" in a more sustained manner. What at first is a series of facts and feelings eventually becomes effortless steadiness with your sun. This is the moving deeper into what is, helping us feel connected and cared for. Or the moon, or a still lake, the sea, the sky, a tree, a flower, a steady flame of light.........That one which you feel a rapport with, which your mind will willingly return to when you find it has strayed to other thoughts, can be your object of meditation.

Perhaps following your own breath as it enters and leaves your nostrils or as your abdomen moves gently is your preference. Or a mantra or chant in your mother tongue that is meaningful to you, at first chanted softly outwardly and then followed silently with the mind and heart. Or align your mantra with your breathing, repeating each line as you inhale and again as you exhale, aligning the rhythm of your words with the comfortable length of your breath. Here is where the definition between breathing practice and mind practice becomes ethereal.

Or holding the feeling of love, of light, of peace, of a divine energy, of the formless, is your homecoming. Or the perennial inquiry 'Who am I?'

In order to generate this positive habit, choose one focus and stay with it over time. Morning helps set the tone for the day ahead; evening helps clear the day's impact and prepares us for deep rest. Begin with a short time each day, moving towards a longer period, and once a day moving towards morning and evening sessions. As with Montessori education, it is our natural curiosity and the love of learning that is the impulse. Even if we just take our 'seat' (which can be a chair) daily to set the stage, even if the mind is at first restless, know that over time the ability and enjoyment will unfold like it has for every other person who has made this choice.

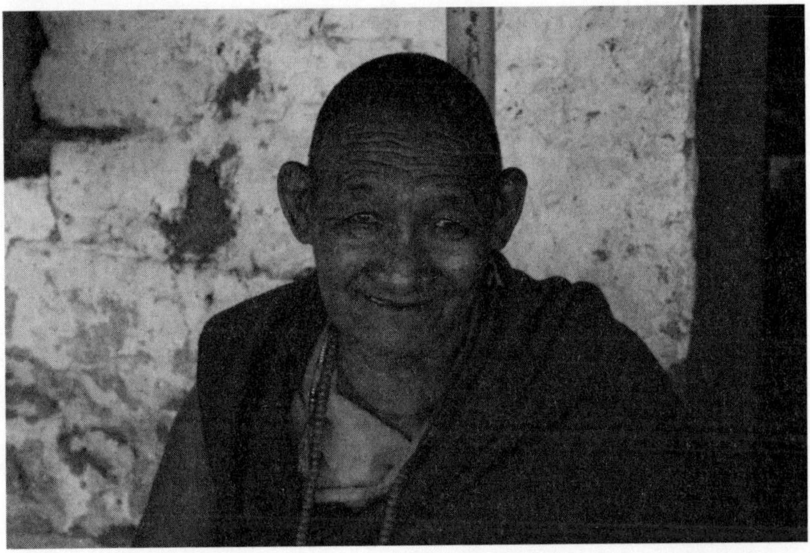

It may still be elusive what we are doing, so let's repeat. Meditation does not mean daydreaming. Then the mind is floating along of its own accord with no one steering. Pleasant as reverie and wishful thinking may be, it doesn't get us anywhere. Nor does it mean rehashing painful history, keeping the past alive and adding to its impact on the present. Bringing the mind from distraction (such as thoughts coming up seemingly without end or the noises around you drawing your mind outward) to direction (deepening the energy pathways where the mind doesn't stray out to everything it could) is the path to meditation. The state of mind called meditation is when even though everything else is as it is, you become so absorbed in your object of meditation these other objects and thoughts disappear from your awareness. You even release your sense of 'I'. The rapport is all there is but if it is named by the mind, it disconnects. If you have ever found yourself so absorbed in the sports page or a good book that you didn't know it until someone says, "Didn't you hear me? I was talking to you!" that is the same ability of the mind to be absorbed. The gap is found between thoughts so a person practiced in meditation experiences the sports page's teams to be part of the one unity, arising and dissolving. As novices, we want our meditation practice to bring us more healing than the contents of the sports page, so we choose a holistic focus.

If you wish, add this meditation time to the end of yoga practice after relaxation. If it is more convenient to sit at another time, slowly phase yourself outward when done, listening, feeling and then opening your eyes.

Equal to good digestion, the teachings of ayurveda state that stress is going to make a good thing go bad. Meditation is the way to reduce mental stress and hence physical stress. Your meditation practice can bring you insights, peace, and understanding. And yet there is nothing we have to achieve. The experience and the effect of the experience is the same thing. Our minds relax, our hearts relax, it seems the space around us has relaxed. Then we go and do and are in the world, and with each day's practice it is through a more expansive, calmer state of mind.

## Weeks 13 & 14 — KICHURI

This basmati rice and split mung bean curry may be the most perfect food there is. It has a low glycemic index, a complete protein profile, has been used in weight-loss nutrition, is tasty and easy to prepare. The energetics are balanced so it is not too heating or cooling and is easy to digest especially with the spices that are included. It provides good bulk in the colon and assists easy elimination. It is sattwic, which means it promotes mental balance. In India it is called bachelor food because men find it easy to cook.

Gather the following ingredients and store them together so that they are easily accessed each time you prepare kichuri.

For each person:

- 1/4 cup basmati rice + 1/8 cup split mung beans

Wash and soak if possible for one hour. Bring to boil in a generous one cup of water. Skim off the foam, add half a teaspoon of grated ginger, cover and simmer for 20-30 minutes. Add water if necessary to keep moist.

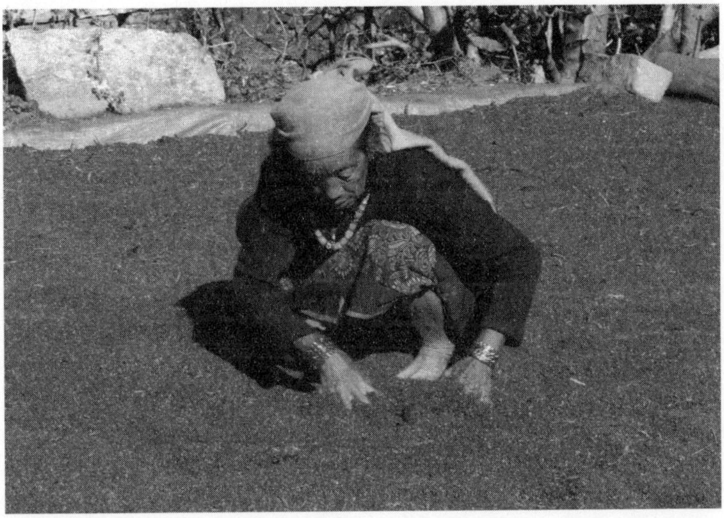

Meanwhile, warm a small skillet over medium heat and add a sprinkle of mustard seed + a sprinkle of cumin seed.

When the first seed pops, remove skillet from heat. Mustard seeds can get bitter if roasted too long. Add 1 teaspoon ghee or oil of choice (not margarine, lard, hydrogenated spreads or GMO oils) and when that dissolves add:

- ¼ teaspoon cumin powder
- ¼ teaspoon coriander powder

- ¼ teaspoon turmeric powder
- ¼ teaspoon Himalayan (rock) salt
- a sprinkle of asafoetida (hing)

The ingredients should sizzle gently in the pan with the residual heat. If they don't, return the skillet to the stove on low heat until they do. Then remove. The grated ginger could be added to the skillet as a variation.

When the rice and mung are almost cooked, add skillet ingredients, mix and finish cooking. Garnish with chopped fresh cilantro (coriander).

Himalayan salt is a mineral-rich earth salt. If you cannot find it use the best salt you can. Substitute quinoa for the split mung as a variation.

During this time, dine on kichuri twice a week. You can make it in the morning and take it in a thermos to work. You can make a double portion and have it for two meals in one day, reheating on the stove top or oven. If you eat kichuri and ama-reducing broth often you will notice the ama on your tongue decreases.

# Weeks 15 & 16 — YOGA

Working without expecting any particular outcome, it is then easy and enjoyable to be with our body and breath as they are.

## PROGRAM B

Blessings on your experience of yoga.

### SITTING

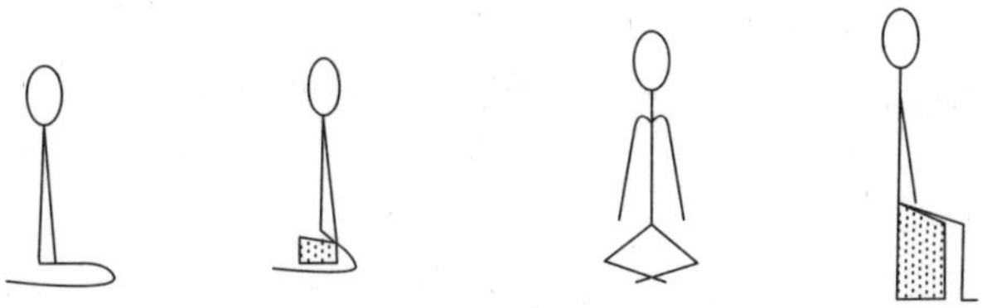

Commence your awareness of breathing in a seated position. Keep your torso comfortable and upright, your face soft. Breathe less rather than more, which, if comfortable and satisfying, will relax you. Yoga can be expressed in the quality of your actions and attention.

### HOBBIT YOGA

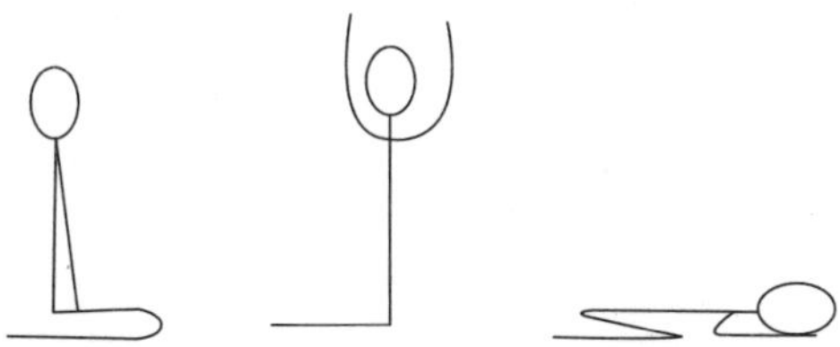

*optional start* *inhale* *exhale*

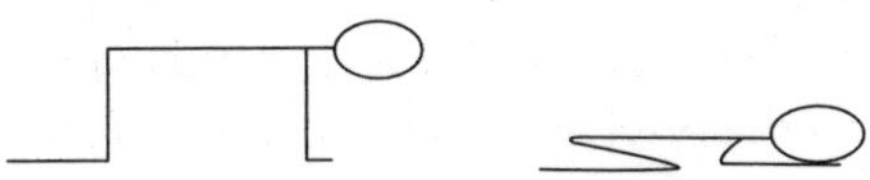

*inhale* *exhale*

This sequence alternates back arches with forward bends. Raising the arms overhead stretches your sides. Raise them only as high as they go easily; your torso remains steady. Avoid dropping too deep into your lower back when on all fours. If you are unable to work on your knees, sit on a chair, alternating arms overhead on inhales as you lift your spine evenly upward and forward bends on exhales, hands moving towards the ground. Let your spine be fluid, long and strong from sitting bones to crown. Move dynamically through the sequence, allowing the breath to begin moving before the body begins moving. Rest for one or two breaths at the end. Do this four times. Please do not force your knees, ankles or back into the child's pose. The outcome of learning the choreography is that the mind merges with the movement of body and breath.

## BHUJANGASANA

"pose of the cobra"

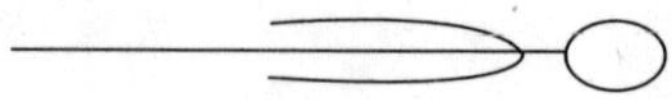

*exhale*

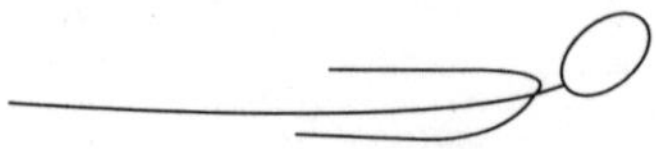

*inhale*

*second variation*

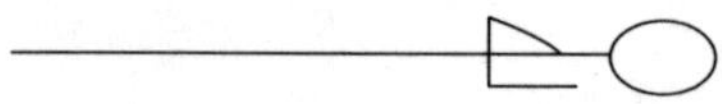

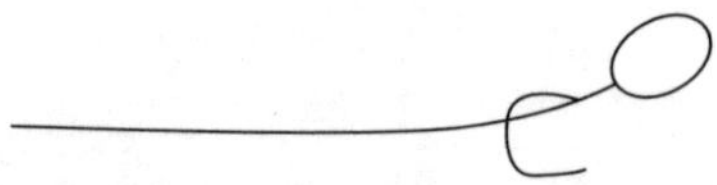

This arch strengthens and makes supple your back. Practice dynamically with the breath initiating the movements four times, then stay up in the pose 4 breaths. Practice both variations. Make sure that you are not levering off your navel to go into the pose and that you are using less and less effort to rise. Cobra will phase out if you are pregnant. You could practice squatting during this part of the program or sitting upright with the soles of your feet touching.

## SITTING TWIST

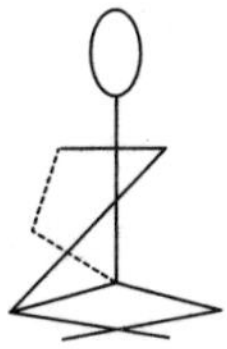

All twists spiral the abdominal area, helping digestion, assimilation and elimination. A *gentle* twist may still be appropriate during pregnancy as it is a natural movement. Choose a seated position. Exhale, twist to the right commencing the twist from the base of your spine; inhale, return to center, base leading, head last. Keep your spine long so that the discs are decompressed. Revolve from side to side for four pairs. Then exhale and start the twist from the top of the spine downward, both sides, four pairs. Did that feel different? There is no right or wrong if it feels safe. Exhale, twist to the right and stay 4 breaths. Inhale, return the torso to center. Exhale, spiral to the left and stay in the pose for 4 breaths. Inhale, return to center.

Lie down. When symmetrical, exhale and once the breath is under way bring your knees over your torso (apanasana). Stay, breathe and enjoy stretching. Then exhale and lower your legs, choosing a supine option and rest for 5 minutes. We practice resting so we can actually do it. Your body becomes soft, open and grounded. The space around you becomes still.

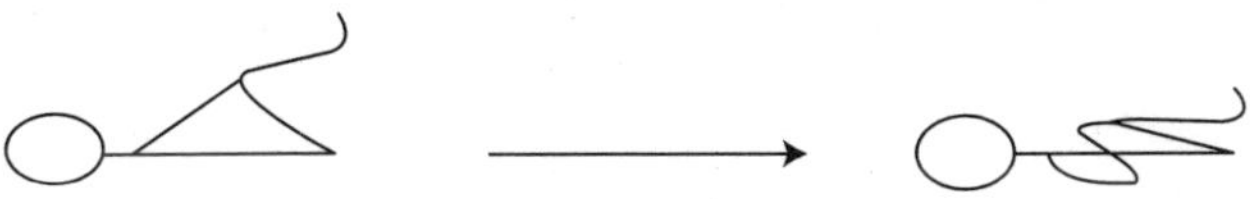

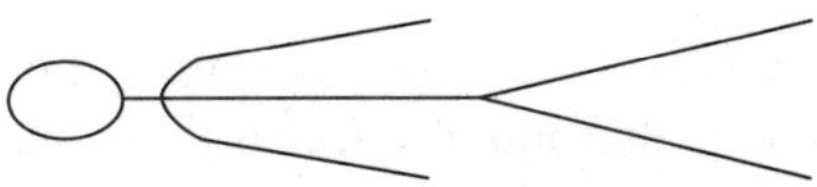

If there is a recognizable difference between how you felt at the beginning and how you feel at the end of Program B, acknowledge it.

Commence Program B and follow with or without Program A three to seven times a week.

# Weeks 17 & 18 —
# NURTURE YOUR DIGESTIVE FIRE

In India, this fire is thought of as a deity to whom we offer oblations. Anything that is taken by mouth, even water, is an oblation and acted on by our digestion. The "fire" consists of enzymes and secretions. All symptoms of indigestion alert us to imbalance. Perhaps what follows will help your digestion. We have already practiced eating freshly cooked foods, ama-reducing broth and kichuri. During these two weeks:

- Eat when hungry
- Don't eat when not hungry
- Eat solid food when hungry rather than drinking a beverage
- Consume beverages at room temperature or warmer
- Eat, seated, in a settled state of mind, body and surroundings
- Eat the largest/heaviest meal around midday
- Moderate alcohol consumption
- Avoid a large or heavy meal late at night
- Avoid overly spicy and overly sour foods
- Avoid overeating or excessive fasting
- Avoid heavy, greasy, leftover foods

Sit for 5 minutes after eating and then walk 108 paces. Keep your abdomen soft in parasympathetic mode for the next hour so you can rest and digest but don't sleep. Ideally you are breathing through your right nostril.

If there is one teaching in ayurveda that stands above all others it is that good digestion, both mental and physical, is the foundation of good health. Leftovers can never be digested properly because the energy of the food has already been transformed by heat. A refrigerator or freezer cannot change this fact. On an ongoing basis eating leftovers leads to foggy thinking, lack of energy, weight gain and degenerative disease. This is a good time to recall that ayurveda contains insights about longevity and that eating freshly cooked food prepared with fresh ingredients is one of them.

## Weeks 19 & 20 — BEVERAGE

On an ongoing basis

FAVOR hot water with ginger powder after meals

REDUCE coffee, tea, hot chocolate

FAVOR 3 cups kettle-boiled water per day

REDUCE iced or chilled beverages

FAVOR herbal teas

REDUCE sugary drinks

FAVOR pure water

REDUCE carbonated drinks

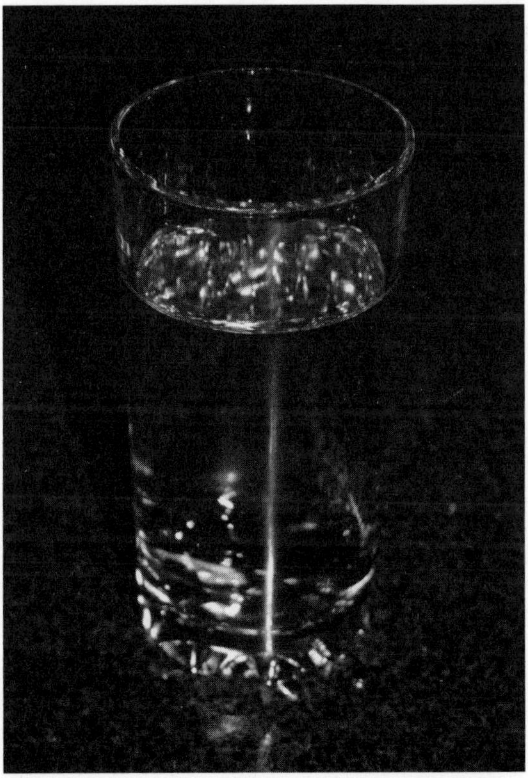

## Weeks 21 & 22 — AMA-REDUCING DIET

Continue to steer your diet in the following way. It is possible to use these two weeks to notice how this could happen and spend the rest of the year putting it in place. It is OK that it takes some serious logistics to get there.

CHOOSE

- fresh foods cooked on the same day
- steamed, baked or sautéed (over low heat) vegetables
- homemade vegetable soups
- well-ripened fruit
- small amounts of chicken (free range), fish or other meats if required
- grains and pulses
- small amounts of best-quality oils

MINIMIZE

- leftovers
- cheese, yoghurt
- fried and oily food
- red meat
- food from a can or jar
- frozen, reheated food
- peanuts and peanut butter
- processed, microwaved and refined foods
- potato, corn chips and anything cooked and packaged
- tea, coffee; any iced or chilled drinks

TREAT YOURSELF to anything your heart desires on occasion.

THE EVENING MEAL needs to be beyond your stomach before you go to sleep. It would be a light cooked meal such as rice, lentils and vegetables or soup and flatbread. Dinnertime is when people gather together and that meal is important yet need not be heavy.

FAVOR well-ripened fruit eaten on its own

MORE THAN cold, heavy, sweet food using refined sugar

FAVOR cooked grains and pulses with homemade sauces

MORE THAN red meat, cheese, bread, onion, pickled foods

FAVOR cooked vegetables

MORE THAN raw foods as the majority of the diet

FAVOR natural products freshly cooked

MORE THAN that which is fried, refined, processed, previously cooked, microwaved and/or packaged

## WHAT ABOUT CRAVINGS?

These will eventually 'give you up' because as ama disappears, cravings disappear. It will be easier to notice a food's effect on your body and mind when there is less ama in the system. Ultimately, the person in balance can eat most anything on occasion without uncomfortable results.

## BETTER ALTERNATIVES

Use milk and natural sweetener if you drink tea or coffee, it softens the bitterness / astringency. Use cardamom in coffee. Cook greens with a little oil and moderate the amount eaten. Too much fiber dries the colon. Lightly toast bread, it makes it less sodden. Look at the shape of your jaw. A strong jaw reflects a higher capacity for digesting meat.

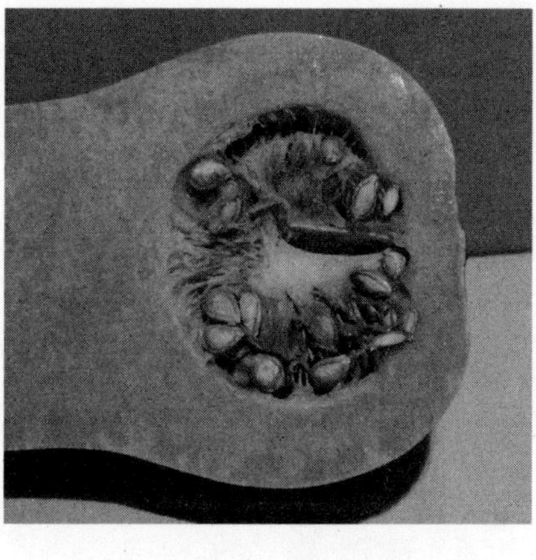

Market

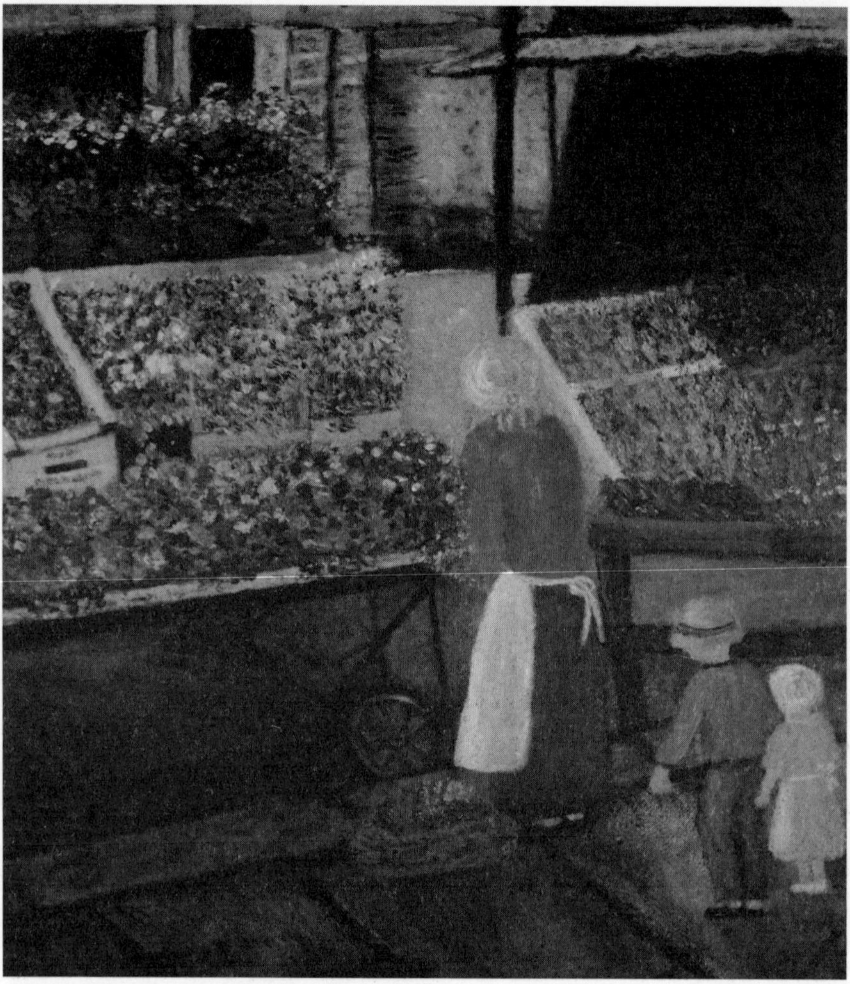

acrylic by Harriet Salem, my mom

# Weeks 23 & 24 — YOGA

Not everyone benefits from a grounded yoga practice. Some people need more activation and standing poses are more active. Smile. Enjoy yourself. Strong and integrated without being stiff, relaxed and spacious without being sloppy. Option: begin with the poses individually and eventually link them in a flow.

## PROGRAM C

Blessings on your experience of yoga.

TADASTHANA / SAMA STHITI

"mountain stance" / "even steadiness"

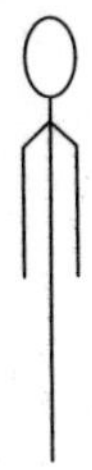

Develop stability, poise, patience, posture and the ability to rest while standing. Also practice whenever you are waiting in line: even tempered body and mind. Even weight between your feet, spine flowing upward, shoulders relaxed, head balanced on your spine. We are already standing on sacred ground.

Commence your breathing awareness. Feel the breath in your whole body, up to your head, down to your feet. When we feel our breath, we may feel connection to that which is in place already as our life, as divine essence breathing us. It happens with chanting too; I am not controlling it yet breath or sound is coming through me.

## UTTANASTHANA

"stretched-out stance"

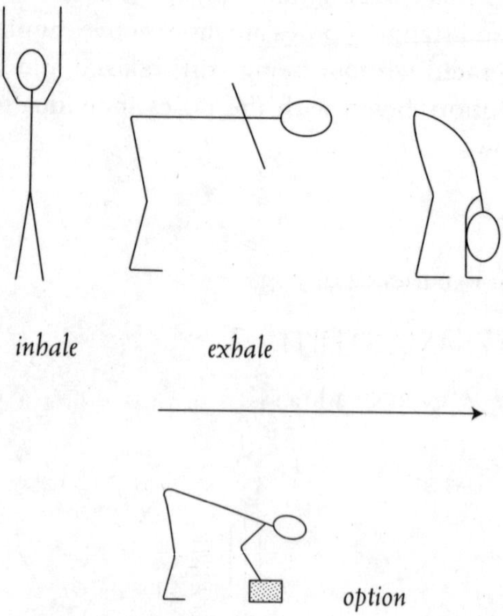


This standing forward bend is a partial inversion. If your blood pressure is above average use the block under your hands so that your head stays more in line with your heart in the horizontal plane. During pregnancy you can widen your stance. Practice dynamically four times with the breath leading each movement. Bending your knees throughout is safest for the spine and spinal cord. Keep your back long and strong (sthira) and relaxed (sukha) simultaneously, the union of which is a description of being in yoga postures. Then stay in the pose for 4 breaths, experiencing the sensations in your body and your breathing. Coming out of the forward bend, your knees are bent, your neck is even, your arms are horizontal and your tailbone moves down and forward to support your lower back on the way up.

## UTKATASTHANA

"intense hip stance"

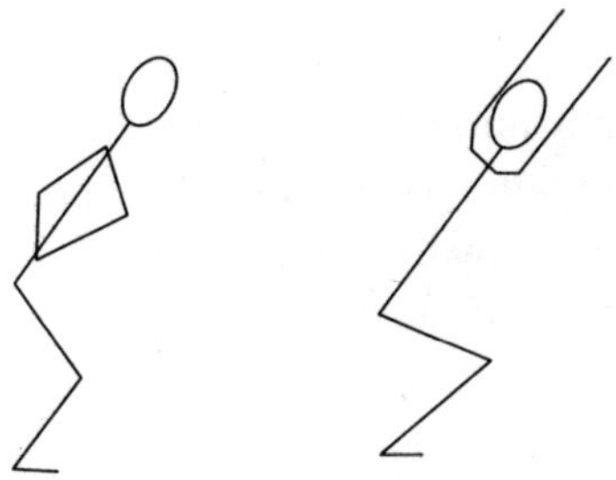

This mobilizes all leg joints and strengthens the body. The second version is strenuous. Make sure your breathing does not become ragged if you practice this version. Please don't make it into endurance training. Notice if your mind wants to do that and if so, smile. Practice the first version dynamically four times: exhale, sit into the chair pose, inhale, stand. Then stay in the pose for 4 breaths. Any place you feel tight is where the energy is not moving. Release as much as possible without losing the strength of the pose. With the second version, inhale, raise your arms, exhale, go into the pose; inhale, return to upright, exhale, lower the arms. Practice four times dynamically, then stay in the pose for 4 breaths. Two leg options: the first is for the feet and legs to be joined together. The second is for them to be hip width apart. In this option make sure your knees move forward rather than knocking together or bowling out.

## TRIKONASTHANA PARIVRITTI

"revolved triangle stance"

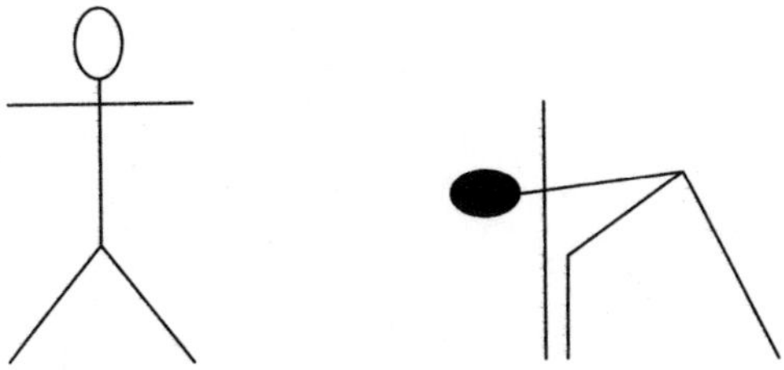

*inhale* *exhale*

This twist and forward bend and partial inversion is done both dynamically led by the breath from side to side, four pairs, and then sustained with 4 breaths each side. One arm is crossed to the opposite leg, the other arm is raised upward or resting, bent at the elbow, on your hip; your face is turned to look upwards or not turned if more comfortable. The knee you are moving towards can bend or both knees can be straight yet not locked. Are you comfortable with the breath leading the movements? It is now the default statement!

To release your body in any further way, include child's pose and/or apanasana. Then lie in supine for 5 minutes. Feel tranquillity spread through you. Serene. Feel clarity spread through you like moonbeams. Lucid. Feel healing spread through you like sunbeams. Radiant.

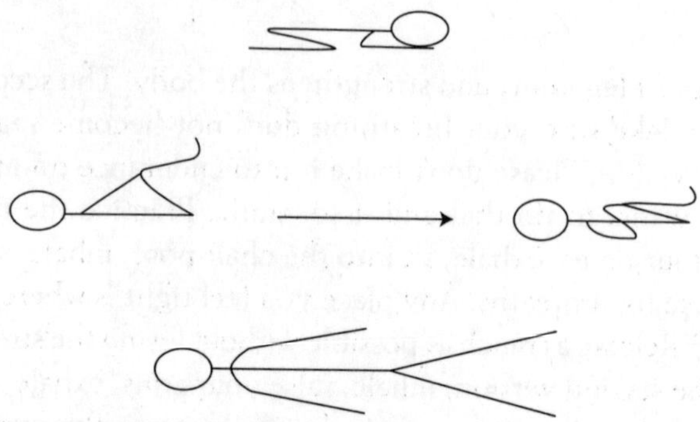

Commence Program C and follow with or without Programs B, then A, three to seven times a week.

# Weeks 25 & 26 — BOWEL CLEANSE

This is a watershed occasion, completing half a year of slowly changing mind, body, habits, energy and awareness. A bowel cleanse is a definitive experience that causes us to take notice. There is something courageous in taking an agent of elimination by mouth that will liquefy the contents of the digestive system and exit the other side. It is a wake-up-shake-down. It is not like a hospital bowel purge. It is much gentler. For some people this is the most confrontational recommendation and for some a bowel cleanse is not a recommendation at all.

Choose an evening when you can stay home the next day. Eat dinner choosing from kichuri, vegetables, vegetable soup and/or flatbread no later than 7 PM. It is best not to eat heavy foods this evening or any evening.

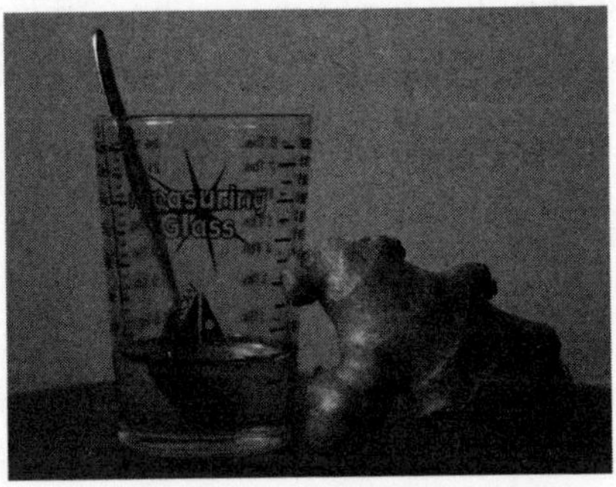


At 10 PM shake 4 level teaspoons of castor oil (20 ml) with 2 teaspoons (10 ml) fresh squeezed ginger juice or orange juice or warm water. To get fresh ginger juice, finely grate the ginger and squeeze it out by hand, then strain. Drink and follow with a cup of warm water. Refined castor oil requires a higher dosage than the unrefined variety. If your colon is very dry (constipation is one indication) even 4 teaspoons of oil will not produce a cleanse as the oil is doing another job, oleating the dryness. In that case take one teaspoon of oil or ghee each evening before bed with warm water for a week prior to trying again.

Go to sleep.

In the morning, or perhaps sooner, you will have several bowel movements which start as semi-solid and become more watery and unformed. If you feel nothing is happening, your morning hot water may activate your system. If feces are small in size or fall apart, or include the passing of air or are dark in color, there is a drying imbalance. If sour in odor and greenish in color with a burning sensation, there is a heat imbalance. If sticky, with mucus and a "sweet" odor, there is a congestive imbalance. Four or more bowel movements indicate a good cleanse. Replace fluid excreted with an approximately equal amount of warm water in the ratio of 1 cup combined with ¼-teaspoon rock or sea salt and 1-teaspoon unrefined sugar. Continue to drink warm water or just the clear broth of the ama-reducing broth. If at any time you wish to stop the cleanse start drinking green tea. When you feel hungry, have the vegetables from the broth or kichuri, or something cooked and easy to digest.

The bowel cleanse clears the body and mind as well. Removing impurities removes their influence on us. Up until the time of your break-fast, your psyche is freeing itself of foreign influence. You rest more and more in your own pristine consciousness.

What happens to a large majority of people at this stage is that they feel drained and blame it on the bowel cleanse and light meals. It is my opinion that what causes the feeling of tiredness is that people are no longer running on nervous energy so they feel how tired the body-mind actually is. This is one of the reasons you keep this day for yourself. We are practicing extended non-doing. Doing can include relaxed walks and contemplations in nature, yoga, easy listening music, reading inspirational books, journaling, painting, writing poetry or prose. Some people get a great rush of energy and clean the house, shed, garden, whatever, like a whirlwind. Don't. Calm yourself, breathe, and let that energy be used for internal housekeeping.

At most, women can do this cleanse each month half a week before their menstrual period. At most, men and women in menopause can do this every three weeks. At most, children from the age of five can begin with ½-teaspoon oil in warm water every few months. Many children do not find this a problem so don't pre-influence them! A monthly cleanse is not recommended for all but is a good thing for most people, helping to remove the impurities we accumulate as a by-product of diet, lifestyle and environment. Notice the recommendation is stated above as "at most". As amazing as this sounds, bowel cleansing can get addictive. Please don't undertake this if you are sick or if your digestion is weak.

Aloe vera juice or gel (certified pure by the International Aloe Council) can be taken orally, 3 teaspoons three times daily before meals. Aloe is a wonder substance that can provide a mild bowel cleanse in those who, for physical considerations, would find a castor oil cleanse too strong. Aloe stimulates the liver prior to eating. If it makes your bowel too loose and you do not want that effect, decrease the amount taken. Aloe is also cooling so consider that effect as well.

Castor oil is especially recommended for people with a strong fiery constitution, those with excess heat in the body or feelings of impatience and anger.

If there is any feeling of cramping you can use massage and warmth over the abdomen.

# Weeks 27 & 28 — HEAD MASSAGE

Abhyanga means all limb total body massage. When someone else does it, which is a great idea, it is called snehana. Sneha means oil, and more oil is used than in abhyanga. It also means friendship and love and the person massaging you should convey that through their heart and hands.

If your skin is dry, performing abhyanga at least every other day is of great benefit. In ayurvedic terms, conditions such as constipation and osteoporosis are signs of excess dryness. This is alleviated with, amongst other things, regular sesame oil massage. If you tend to be overwrought, massage is a good way to center and calm down. If you drift into lethargy, a massage can stimulate your system.

Apply some sesame oil or coconut oil to the inside of your nostrils with your most comfortable finger pad, gently, not too deeply, with a trimmed nail. This keeps the passages oleated and can help prevent allergies. Apply several times a day especially in dry, cold, hot or windy climates.

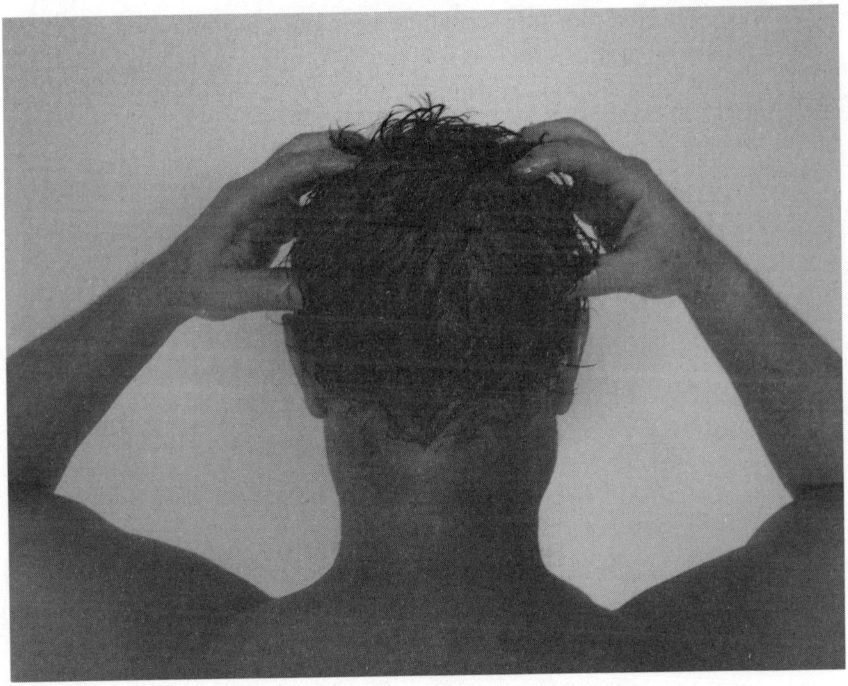

## THE MASSAGE

1. Transfer one teaspoon of warm oil from the palm of your hand to your crown in a circular movement as a blessing. Apply about three more teaspoons to various areas of your scalp and massage in circular movements and moving the skin of the scalp over the bone of the skull. Your massage would include the base of your skull, hairline and ears. Coconut oil is the general choice for head massage.

2. Leave on overnight, covering your pillow with a towel. You can wear a beanie if you feel your head is getting too cold. By now your family is no longer surprised by the things you do and is maybe doing them too. How could a family of beanies not enjoy themselves?

3. Scalp massage is good for the sinuses, brain, sense organs and mind. It is also good for hair growth and scalp health.

4. Wash out next morning with mild shampoo. In India there are herbal preparations such as soap nut and shikakai that are used instead of shampoo. Sudsing is not seen as the indicator of cleansing. Wash out sooner if desired.

5. Do this twice to three times a week for these two weeks and then once or twice a week thereafter.

# Weeks 29 & 30 — CHANTING in ENGLISH

Tall Trees - Lyrics by Tony Wrench, Arrangement by Graham Russell-Pead used with permission.

Find a comfortable place to sit. Chanting sets up an internal vibration. It reaches every cell. Let the vibration be healing.

Either read the music below or make up your own melody.

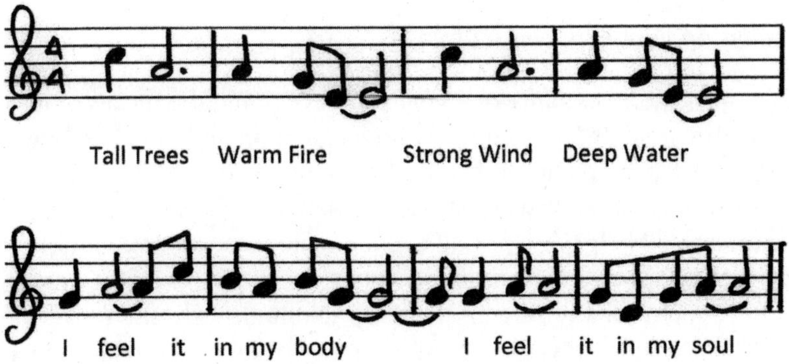
Tall Trees Warm Fire Strong Wind Deep Water
I feel it in my body I feel it in my soul

## WITH VOWEL AND SEMI-VOWEL SOUNDS

Instead of using the words, use the following sounds, one time through the melody with each sound.

Ah (short a); AA (long a); Ee; Oh; Oo; R; L; M.

## TALL TREES LULLABY

Change the original words to the following, one time through the melody with each phrase. Once you get the idea, create a song relevant to you and your family that you can sing together. It can be serious or silly - laughing is such a great practice.

Mama; Papa; Yes, dear; Can't sleep; What to do; Sing to me; Which song; Tall Trees; ~and now sing the actual song~

# Weeks 31 & 32 — YOGA

If our bodies had different limbs that worked in a different way, an alternate form of torso, neck and head, and if we did not breath as we do, our practice would be different! When we participate in these postures we are united with what is given: our bodies as they are, life in this form on this planet with its elements, in this sun system, in this universe. That is yoga.

## PROGRAM D

Blessings on your experience of yoga.

Yoga is also the assembling of a goal and developing the means of moving towards the goal. It is gaining new understanding and novel abilities. For example, if a person cannot do the following pose, they would consider what the pose is about and perhaps find different ways of experiencing that. A teacher could help. Or a person could practice with baby steps until their body acclimated to the experience. One of the beauties of yoga postures is that they engage many parts of the body simultaneously and move energy from high pressure areas to low pressure areas. Yoga is not corralling ourselves into fixed patterns of thinking, or feeling obligated to do something "right". It is about exploring how we are and feeling comfortable with ourselves. Instructions are guidelines.

Begin by sitting or lying, centering and commencing your yoga breathing.

### ADHO MUKHA SVANASANA

"down-faced dog pose"

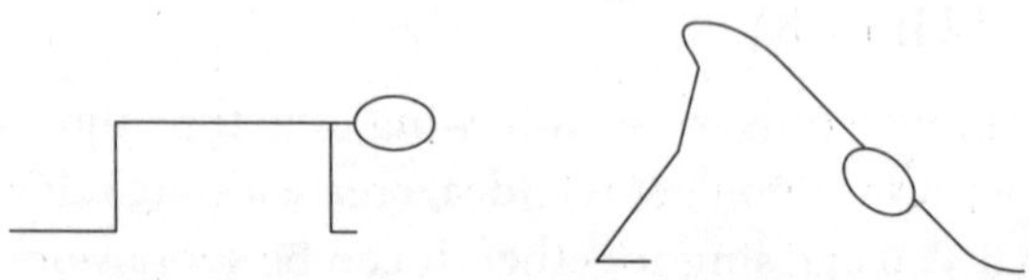

This pair moves from all fours to the dog pose. It is a partial inversion. Inhale while on all fours. Exhale, move into the pose. Inhale in the pose and exhale, move back to all fours. Inhale there. Practice this dynamically four times and then stay in down dog for 4 breaths. Remember to let the movement of breath begin before the larger physical movements.

## SURYA NAMASKAR

"salutation to the sun" variation

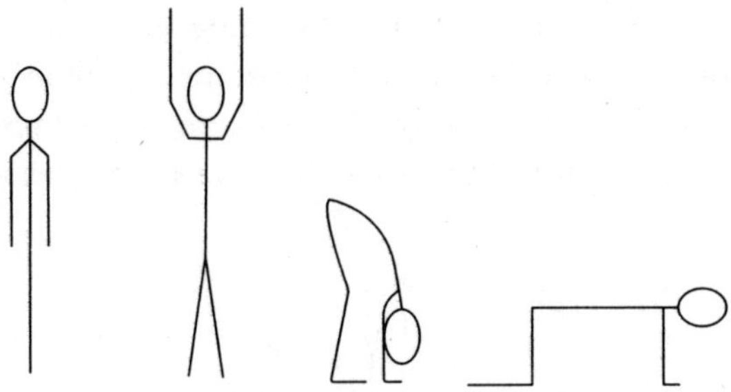

*sama sthiti* *inhale* *exhale* *inhale*

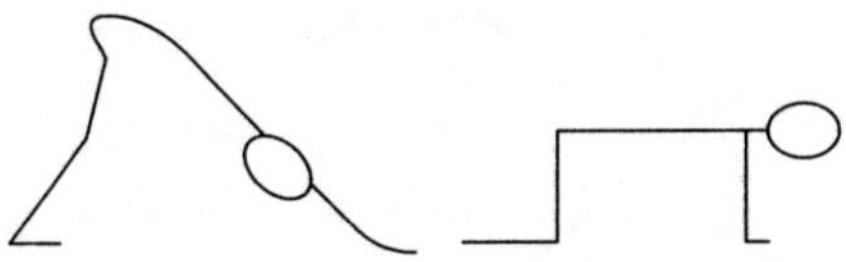

*exhale* *inhale*

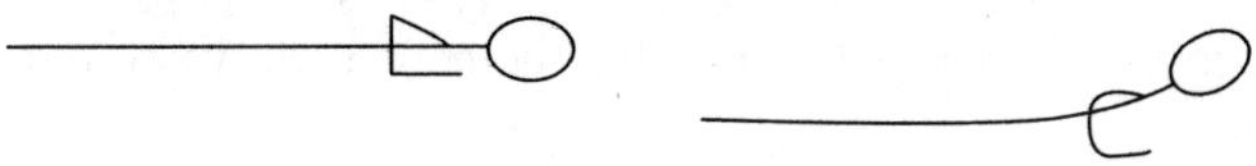

*exhale* *inhale*

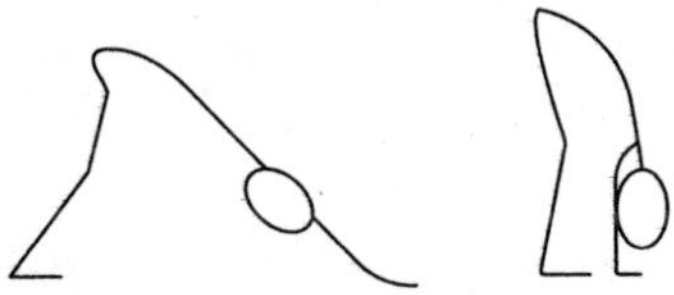

*exhale* *inhale and exhale*

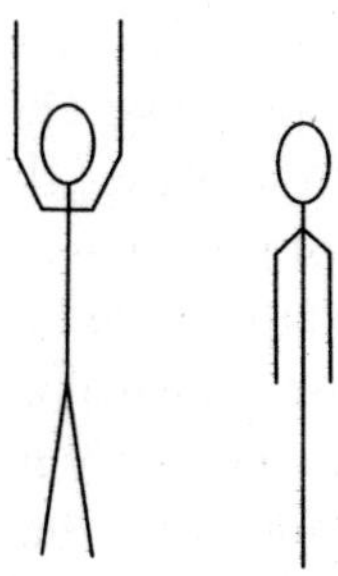

*inhale* *exhale*

It is traditional to face the rising sun to practice Surya Namaskar. Repeat several times dynamically. If the breathing suggestions do not feel right for you, please change them. If in doubt, exhale going into a pose. If your breathing gets discordant, you may be using your energy rather than generating more. You may be making it more aerobic than yogic and that's OK if that is your choice. It is possible to use yoga postures aerobically or as dance moves. Yoga provides ease and breathing awareness while moving.

## SITTING TWIST

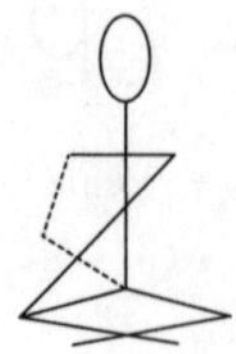

Practice this twist as suggested in Program B. Or make up a new version or try humming while exhaling. Mmmmmmmmm.............

As you lie down practice apanasana, stretching both sides of your back evenly. Then rest in supine for 5 minutes, experiencing how simple things can be when your body is resting after your work in work out and your mind is quiet.

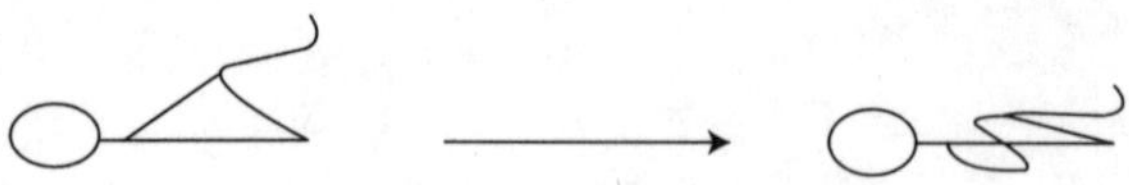

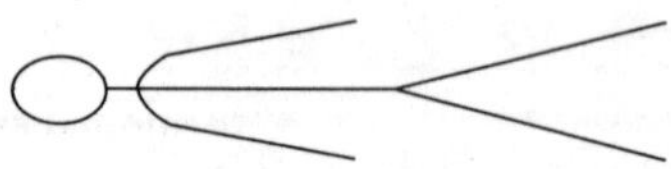

BREATHING while sitting up gives the most freedom to the diaphragm and rib cage and the most mental alertness. The extended, delicate, smooth breath calms the nervous system and uses the diaphragm as the central muscle it is while using all parts of the lungs. It is most important that you feel ease and comfort when regulating your breath. The direction we head in is to breathe less and less while feeling calm. Breathing less helps extend longevity because even though we need oxygen, oxygen oxidizes us away. If we allow carbon dioxide to accrue in our bloodstream as we breathe less, it opens the bronchi and the blood vessels so that oxygen reaches the cells more efficiently. It also causes us to eat a more alkaline diet. However, we live in the present experience, rather than the future-not-yet-experience so enjoy breathing in whatever way you breathe. While the yoga postures are primarily for the body, they assist with focusing the mind; breathing practices are used primarily to decrease the blippy movements of the mind and the body needs to be comfortable. We cannot grasp the mind as an object so we work on its function through our breath. Movement of breath and movement of mind are two sides of the same coin. One of the reasons people experience increased ease in life when they practice yoga is because of this effect of the breath.

Try this with book in hand: GROUND, feel your natural breath for awhile. ONE, breathe with soft pelvic floor, as if breathing just from there. Take several breaths with this. TWO, feel the lower abdomen open gently with the inhale and release gently with the exhale. Breathe until you really connect with it. THREE, if you know the ujjayi sound, include that for several more breaths. Ujjayi gives an audible reference to the length and smoothness of breathing. Let it be audible to mainly just you, that is, not loud or forceful.

FOUR, notice that as you exhale, the abdomen naturally moves somewhat toward your spine. Allow a brief pause after exhaling. As you begin to inhale let the collarbones lift and widen rather than the abdomen inflate. Towards the end of the inhale, allow the abdomen to be relaxed without being distended and allow softness in your sides. Please don't over-inflate or over-deflate your lungs, that will just produce tension. Allocate a brief pause after the inhale too. Breathe another several with this awareness.

This pattern is based on the teachings of Sri T. Krishnamacharya. The breath moves to and from the spine, the breath moves the spine. If you are comfortable with ujjayi breathing combined with spinal breathing, continue for more breaths, as many as you like. Then release the spinal breathing and be with THREE, ujjayi with soft belly a few breaths; then release the ujjayi and be with TWO, soft belly for a few breaths; then release the belly breathing and ONE, breathe into the base of your body. Now GROUND, let the body breathe by itself and turn your attention to dharana.

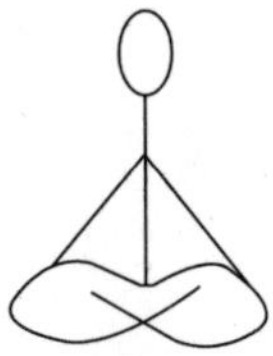

DHARANA is forming a mental relationship with an object or concept that pleases you. We come to reflect and be the qualities of our object of contemplation. I offer here a form of meditation, contemplation of Krishnamacharya's teachings (India, 1888-1988). Consider the meaning of these words in your life:

Regulate the Breath

Be Happy

Link the Mind with the Divine in Your Heart

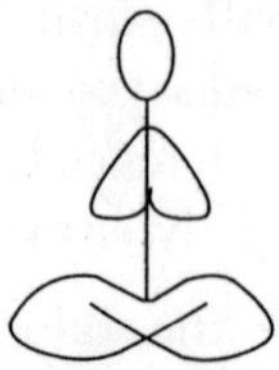

*om shanti*
*om peace*

Commence Program D three to seven times per week. Commence using ujjayi spinal breathing (see FOUR above) in all yoga postures from now on, if comfortable. If you wish to form a complete practice of all the programs, begin with the postures in Program D, then C, then B, then A. Resting for one minute between programs is adequate. After a full rest following Program A, return to the Breathing and Dharana of Program D. Sweet.

# Weeks 33 & 34 — FORGIVE and FORGET

Our internal mental environment, where we live in our minds, how we think and feel, is the one aspect that is most powerful in its effect on our wellbeing. Psychoimmunoneuroendocrinology is the study of the chemicals we produce with our thoughts and feelings that are circulated to all parts of the body and affect our health. We don't just live in our heads. Several times a day during these two weeks tell your body with your thoughts and feelings that "We're good." Find a thought and feeling that makes that an honest statement. Relax those areas of your body where your mental fretting makes them contract.

Ayurveda encourages our practice of selfless service, unconditional love, forgiving and forgetting. Through meditation, prayer, placing a ceiling on desires, good deeds, and self-reflection, we will experience better health. All of this is about you, about the flavor and nature of the fluids circulating within you.

Of the recommendations in this book, massage, yoga, meditation and a pure diet are gateways to emotional and mental balance.

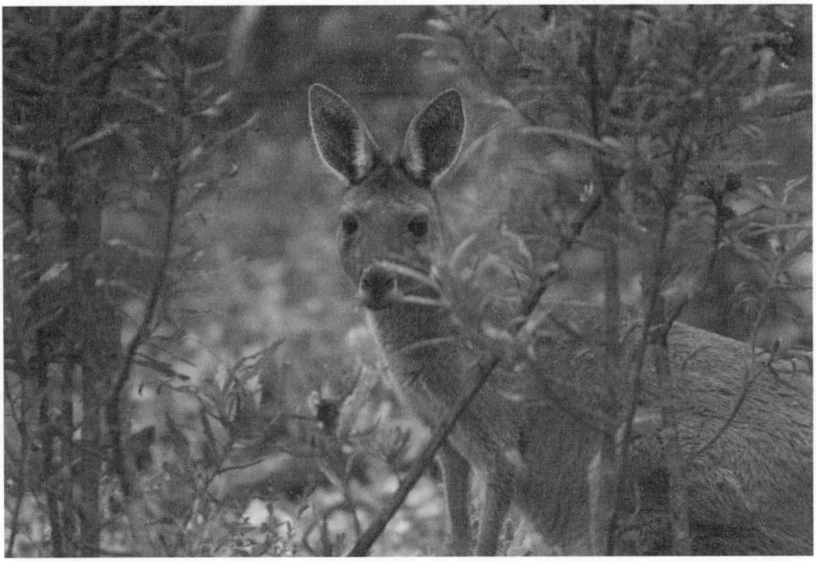

# Weeks 35 & 36 —
# BREATHING and MEDITATION

Prepare your yoga relaxation area.

**Begin** sitting with the following breathing meditation by Thich Nhat Hanh.

**Think to yourself and feel as you inhale**: "Breathing in, I know I am breathing in."

**Think to yourself and feel as you exhale**: "Breathing out, I know I am breathing out." Do this for several breaths and then shorten the phrases to "In." "Out."

**Second phase**: "Breathing in, my breath grows deep." "Breathing out, my breath grows slow." This becomes "Deep." "Slow."

**Third phase**: "Breathing in, I feel calm." "Breathing out, I feel ease." This becomes "Calm." "Ease."

**Fourth**: "Breathing in, I smile." "Breathing out, I release." "Smile." "Release."

**Fifth**: "Breathing in, I dwell in the present moment." "Breathing out, I know it is a wonderful moment." "Present moment." "Wonderful moment."

Stay as many breaths as you wish with each phase. Please feel what the words are saying rather than just saying the words. Your brain will then be in alpha wave mode and can merge into your meditative practice.

Or switch on a guided meditation recording such as yoga nidra and lie down slowly and evenly as you do in supine, perhaps with a cover over you. Let the voice guide you. Or consider creating your own experience. It could start in a place that appeals to all your senses in which you feel connected and safe. Imagine yourself there in a laboratory of discovery (and you create the machines you need), in a repository of insight and wisdom (and you type in-think in what you want to know), in a place of joy, a haven, a temple (where you are surrounded by and imbued with spirit - people, chanting, prayer).

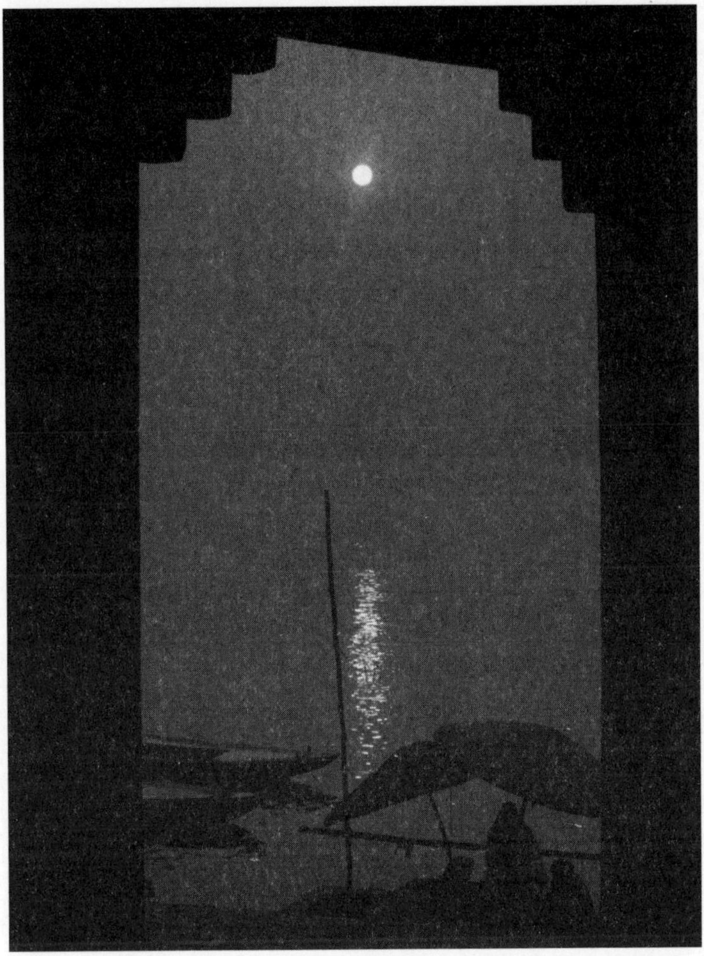

Repeat this during the next two weeks, no less than once a week. If you found that you fell asleep, practice at a different time of day or in a sitting position.

# Weeks 37 & 38 —
# UPGRADE YOUR BOWEL CLEANSE

We now soften and loosen the ama in the body one week prior to the cleanse. For women it is ideal to do this so that it is completed a few days prior to your menstrual period. In that way most of the ama has been eliminated. Then the menstrual period completes the monthly cleanse. If these two weeks do not include that time of your moon cycle, extend this recommendation for another week or two so that it does.

FOR THE WEEK PRIOR TO THE CLEANSE, MEN AND WOMEN:

1. Resume ama-reducing broth twice a day, kichuri, vegetable soups, small amounts of well-reared chicken if necessary and ripe fruit eaten apart from the rest of the meal. Notice that this is a light, cooked diet (with the exception of the fruit and a small amount of raw salad). This will allow the body to extend its energy towards digesting ama rather than digesting food. If you suspect you have candida, worms, flagellates, etc., delete the fruit and hence the sugar.

2. Perform abhyanga every day to move the ama back towards the digestive system to be eliminated. Perform a head massage every other day to soothe the nervous system.

3. Practice yoga, whichever program you wish, everyday.

4. Continue to drink hot water and reduce other beverages.

5. If oral hygiene has lapsed, clean your tongue and do gandush once or twice a day.

6. If you feel that you need a teaspoon of castor oil or ghee in warm water each evening prior to the cleanse, please have it.

Proceed with the cleanse as outlined in weeks 25 and 26. Spend the next day resting as before. Notice if your mind is clearer and more peaceful. It may be that all the recommendations thus far have contributed to that already.

An alternative purgative is magnesium oxide sold as ColoZone or Colon Cleanse. At 10 PM stir 2 level teaspoons into a glass of warm water or freshly squeezed juice. This powder does not dissolve but suspends in the water. Drink this. Squeeze ¼-cup fresh lemon juice and put into the glass with more water, swilling up the remaining powder and drink. Have another glass of warm water if you wish. Go to bed. There may be more noise in your intestines this time as the oxygen gets liberated from the magnesium by the acidic lemon juice.

## Weeks 39 & 40 — RE-INVENTING A RECIPE

Let's take the recipe for hoomus and enliven it. The recipe ingredients are marked with an asterisk.

**BASIC**: 2 cups canned chickpeas or store-bought hoomus.

***SUPERIOR**: Soak 1-cup chickpeas 8 hours and discard water. Add fresh water and cook covered until tender, at least 60 minutes, skimming foam off the top.

**BASIC**: 2 cloves garlic.

***SUPERIOR**: Garlic is a medicine, not to be used casually. Add it occasionally in winter. Add a sprinkle of compounded asafoetida instead.

**BASIC**: Reconstituted lemon juice.

***SUPERIOR**: 2-4 tablespoons fresh lemon or other citrus juice to taste.

**ACCEPTABLE**: 3 tablespoons tahini.

***SUPERIOR**: Use 3 tablespoons freshly dry-roasted sesame seeds ground with hot water or added without grinding.

**BASIC**: 1-teaspoon salt.

***SUPERIOR**: Start with ½-teaspoon rock or sea salt. Too much salt has dulled our palates.

***ADD**: Water or cooking liquid to blend if needed. Sesame or olive oil to garnish. A small amount of oil is a necessary ingredient because it stokes the digestive fire. Always use cold-pressed oils.

***IN ADDITION**: Use 1-teaspoon cumin powder to make the beans more digestible. It is favorable for everyone's use. Experiment with a small amount of fresh ground black pepper as another pungent taste.

### NOTES:

Spices and herbs: experiment with 1-teaspoon mustard seed and 1- teaspoon cumin seed sautéed in 1-teaspoon ghee or oil and added instead of cumin powder. Experiment with paprika, coriander or ajwan. We use their tastes for flavor and to enhance our digestive fire and food digestibility. Not all spices are favorable for everyone. See my cookbook Sattwa Café for more information about aligning recipes to ayurvedic principles.

Respect the service you are performing by cooking. It has been said that we are genetic material, DNA, wrapped in food. Choose only fresh ingredients, freshly cooked. (Has the reader read that sufficiently by now?) Tempering seeds and spices in ghee or oil (sautéing over low heat) makes them more potent. Consider the effect the meal will have on the five senses. Cook and eat with gratitude and remember to rinse your mouth and take a stroll afterwards to assist digestion.

# WEEKS 41 & 42 — CHANTING in SANSKRIT

Honoring the mother as she expresses as the manifest, honoring the father as all possibility, formless. Since the father represents the potential to create, we chant to the mother as the expression of creation in her many forms throughout history, throughout the world. To compose a chant, use words that are meaningful to you and a melody that you like. I composed Jai Maa Shakti myself. Feel free to use it in any application that has heart and soul. At the launch of this book we chanted it and it is posted on youtube as Ayurveda and Chanting.

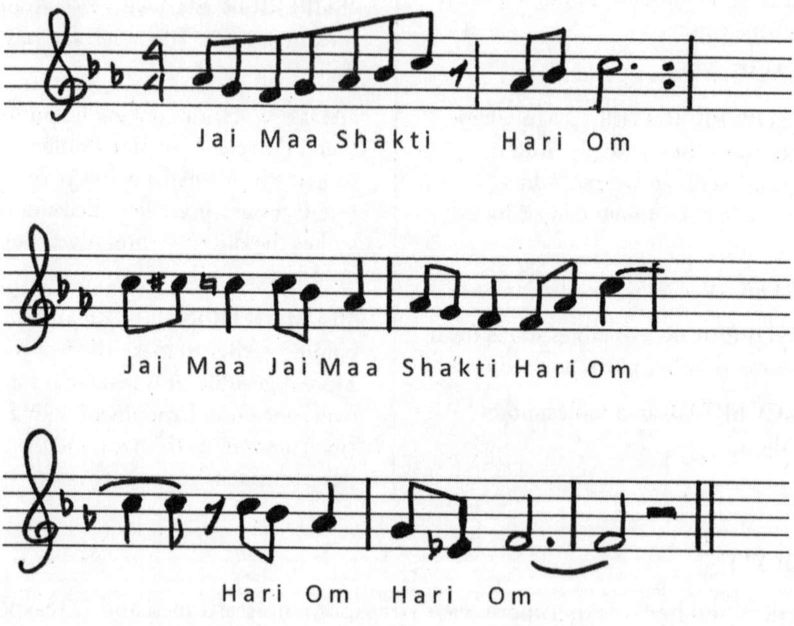

Jai Maa Shakti Hari Om
Jai Maa Jai Maa Shakti Hari Om
Hari Om Hari Om


Instead of the word Shakti which symbolizes all energy as the Great Goddess, use the following images of the Divine Feminine in the chant, one name or more each time through, as many as you wish to name each time you practice this chant. These names are in several languages from several cultures. Complete the chant with names of choice. How about yours or the women in your life?

**Bahuba**
(Zaire, Mother Goddess)

**Epona**
(Celtic, Saxon, Goddess of Horses of the Iron Age)

**Selket**
(Egypt, Scorpion Goddess)

**Aphrodite**
(Greece, Goddess of Love)

**Mary**
(Christian, Divine Mother)

**Shekina**
(Kabala, Primordial Energy of Visible Form)

**Kali**
(India, Goddess who Devours Time)

**Uzuma**
(Japan, Goddess of Merriment)

**Brigid**
(Irish-Gaelic, The Exalted One)

**Mensa**
(Roman, Goddess of Measurement)

**Ariadne**
(Crete, Goddess of the Moon)

**Al-Mah**
(Persia, Goddess of the Moon)

**Zochiquetzal**
(Mexico, Goddess of All Women)

**Freya**
(Norse, Goddess of Love)

**Ixchel**
(Mayan, Goddess of Earth, Moon and Medicine)

**Laima**
(Lithuanian, Goddess of Fortune)

**Hina**
(Polynesia, the Creatress)

**Inanna**
(Sumeria, Queen of Land, Heaven and Moon)

**Ishtar**
(Assyria, Babylon, Goddess of the Hearth, Light of the World)

**Zorya**
(Russia, Triple Goddess of Dawn, Twilight and Midnight)

**Annapurna**
(Nepal, Tibet, Goddess of Perfection, Food)

**Kwan Yin**
(China, Boundless Compassion)

**Edda**
(Norse, Mother Earth)

**Isis**
(Egypt, Female of the Throne, Mortal Woman)

**Pele**
(Pacific, Goddess of Fire, the Volcano, Dance, Lightning, the Underworld)

**Gaia**
(Greece, Earth Goddess)

**Sophia**
(Greece, Goddess of Wisdom)

**Saraswati**
(India, Goddess of Wisdom)

**Rhea**
(Aegean, Universal Mother)

**Diana**
(Roman, Celtic, Goddess of the Moon, the Hunt and Wild Creatures)

**Aditi**
(India, Mother of the Gods)

**Anima-Vegeta-Minera**

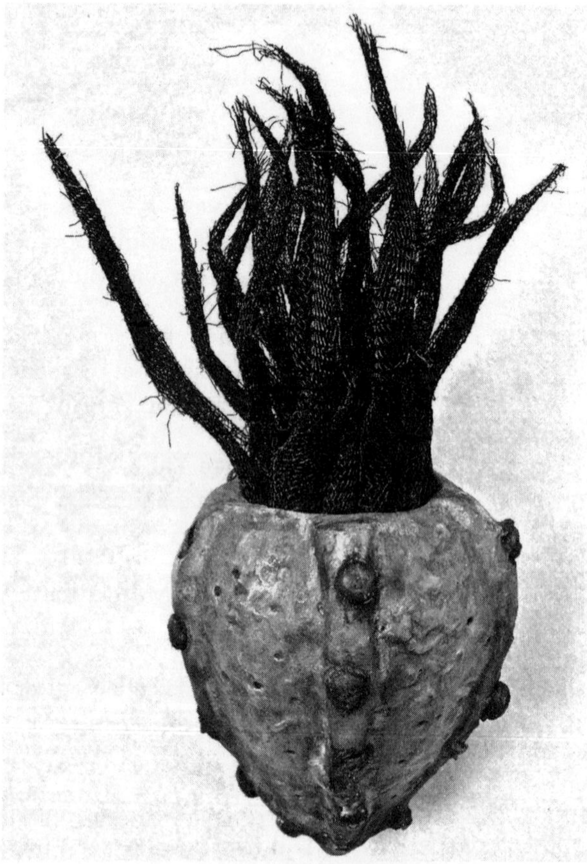

**mixed media by Helen Robins**

# WEEKS 43 & 44 — GENDER HEALTH

To maintain healthy reproductive tissue, organs and fluids we insure that the intrinsic value of the foods we eat is high, that we support the strength of our digestive and metabolic fire and that we take steps to decrease ama which blocks proper nutrient flow, tissue function and even its own elimination. Decreasing stress and worry is important and honoring our partner is too. Ayurveda has a complete limb of knowledge pertaining to reproductive health and what compromises fertility.

Reproductive tissue receives the highest essence of the diet thus indicating how nature has an investment in continuing our species. If the diet is of poor quality and/or if our digestive fire is sluggish or weak and/or if ama is present, we may experience imbalance in this area. Combine that with lifestyle excess and the state of our environment (water, air, indoor chemicals), it is not hard to understand why many couples experience infertility. But that may be just a current imbalance. Many couples have conceived with the help of ayurveda.

Continue living the ayurvedic recommendations and consider the following.

## MALES

- Frequency of emission, however voluntary, depletes this tissue and lowers ojas, our overall natural immunity. Semen is a type of ojas for sperm, cushioning and nutritive. It takes the body 35 days to convert food and energy into sperm. Bestow this tissue the same consideration as nature does.
- Retention of ejaculation and sex while under the influence of various substances can also cause reproductive disorders.
- The use of chemical spermicides may adversely affect both partners' health.
- Allow only natural fibers such as silk or cotton next to your skin and wear loose-fitting underwear and trousers. Did rock stars have fertility problems?
- There are ayurvedic herbs, foods (almonds, dates, ghee, black gram lentils) and massage points to use if sexually active.
- There are yoga postures that benefit the energy of the lower body. Sitting or lying with the soles of the feet together circulates energy in this region.

- A good time for sexual merging is about 9 PM so that the body can re-build its ojas during sleep.

## FEMALES

- Menstruation is purification and a renewal of all metabolisms each month. The seed has experienced its natural end and you are preparing for rebirth, new growth. What mental seeds will now be sown?

- How a woman lives her life during the month is reflected in the experience of the menstrual period. Defying the cycles of nature (day, night, eating, sleeping, working, resting) or if any normal function is impaired, there will be signs of imbalance in the pre-menstrual and menstrual times. We tend to blame menstruation for the symptoms when actually it is lifestyle and diet that are causing the imbalance. See Part Three, Mother and Child Health.

- It is of great importance to rest during the menstrual period because the body is cleansing. Both blood and emotional impurities are released at this time. If we are stressed or physically active we mitigate the efficiency of the cleanse and this will affect the next menses. Do not schedule anything mentally challenging or physically strenuous and request that others prepare the meals. Even yoga and similar practices should be paused at this time. A short walk is beneficial.

- It is also necessary to eat foods that can be digested easily during menses. All physical and physiological functions decrease in strength except for the function of menstruation.

- Pause sexual activity and use pads instead of tampons to support apana, which is responsible for downward movements. When industry and advertising finally get it, we will not be driven to exercise at this time and will still use their products.

- Continue your meditation practice as this is an occasion of great insight and connection to spirit. Mentally release all unhealthy thoughts and feelings and prepare an unbiased field for the next lunar cycle. Because females are greatly influenced by the moon, be aware of its phases.

- The closer we come to natural contraception the healthier we remain. We also ensure the continuity of healthy offspring through what we have put into our own bodies.

- There is a traditional teaching in ayurveda that says that for healthy female organs a woman needs to embrace her birthright as a woman and mother. If not the latter, then at least don't think that your female functions and feminine side are a nuisance. There is mounting popular evidence coming up to speed with traditional teachings that state that menstruation is a blessing, not a curse.

- With menopause the ovarian cycle ends and our hormone balance and health are exquisitely supported through inbuilt pathways as long as we do not encumber them with poor diet or demanding lifestyle.

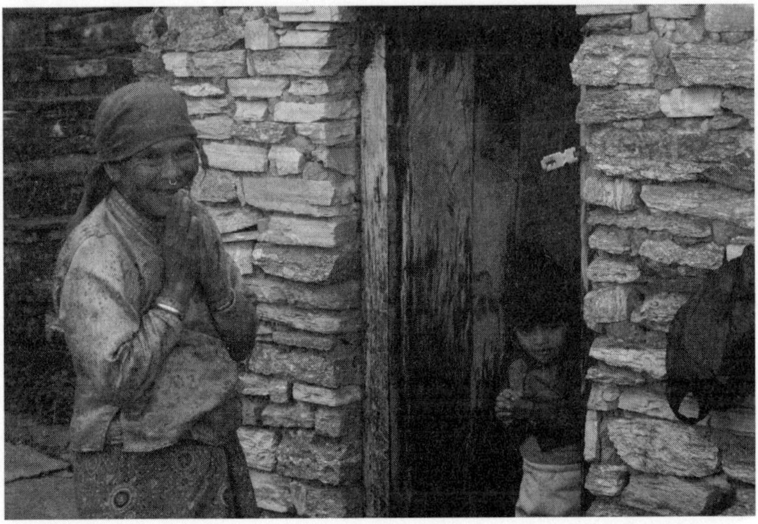

At this stage of life women are wise and more deeply connected to the source of all things. This wisdom would include the first-hand experience of how to take care of themselves so that minimal stress and ama are produced. Without the menstrual period to cleanse the blood, it is more important to foster complete digestion and a healthy lifestyle. Imbalances are more apparent and indicate without question which elements need pacifying. Please refer to the table in Part Three, Mother and Child Health. Hormone production and effectiveness are equated with mental stability: do your meditation practice!

- *Aloe barbadensis*, the gel or juice that you may have been taking called aloe vera from weeks 25 and 26, is a female reproductive tonic and overall liver tonic for everyone. It also helps heal burns, rashes, acne, insect bites and wounds and reduces itching, and helps scrape ama from the small intestines. To ease pre-menstrual, menopausal and hysterectomy symptoms women can take up to 5 teaspoons before meals with a small amount of ginger powder added. This helps ease congested liver, which can help alleviate the symptoms. We pause aloe during pregnancy, lactation, menstruation, hemorrhage or uterine bleeding.

- The Sanskrit name for aloe is kumari, meaning 'she who possesses a thousand husbands'. Feel free to take the energy without that many menfolk.

- With any medicinal herb it is recommended to have a time of non-use so that the body does not habituate to it. These are herbs and spices that one would not add casually to a meal.

For women already on a spiritual path, these recommendations make such perfect sense that they already follow the suggestions or will make the changes with a feeling of AH, YES. For women who are drawn into excessive outward living these ideas will be considered anathema to freedom (what? rest? miss out on life? can't, won't). However, I have never met a woman who doesn't applaud getting someone else to cook during her period.

# WEEKS 45 & 46 — WALKING MEDITATIONS

## WE ARE FROM THIS PLANET

Go outside and use your senses one by one to take in a glorious aspect of the natural world, which that sense brings to you. For instance, have a good look at one color, form, etc. that is pleasant. Have a good listen to one sound that you like. Find an aroma that you know is pleasing and breathe it. Touch something, feel a texture, with full awareness. Perhaps find something edible that you like the taste of and pay attention to that taste. Feel a sense of the environment you are in and how your senses and mind bring that to you. Celebrate your sense of enjoyment through your senses with what the planet offers. Use words, feelings and movements.

Come to a seated position, either outside or inside and immerse yourself in your recollection and the feeling that it creates.

## BE FROM ANOTHER GALAXY

On the same day or on another day go outside and pretend that all you take in through your senses is new to you. Describe something you see with words, thoughts and feelings so carefully that your words, thoughts and feelings translate like a living experience for others in your galaxy. As an omniversal being there is no judgment. This being would not say the plant looks ragged and smells bad (careful with allergies, earthling). It would notice the way the edges of the leaves appear and its aroma. Do this for each sense. It is unbiased description we are with here, keeping the mind from inserting labels such as like/dislike, nice/not nice, etc.

Come to a seated position and flow with this light feeling, open to input without value qualification. This meditation can also be done walking along, where we just look, listen, smell and feel. Notice when you have lapsed into opinion and let go, becoming more aware of the habits of the mind and how often they arise.

Practice these two meditations several times each week.

# WEEKS 47 & 48 — OTHER RECOMMENDATIONS

Ayurveda recognizes 6 basic tastes: sweet, salty, sour, pungent, bitter and astringent. A meal should be a blend of these tastes. The sweet taste is predominant in all foods and the rest are condiments. We usually use some salt (salty) and pepper (pungent). Sometimes we squeeze on some lemon juice (sour) and astringency is in all fruit and vegetables, especially green leaves. That leaves bitter which most people steer clear of and yet it is light and detoxifying. Here's where the aloe is a good addition, as an aperitif. Ayurveda spice powder blends can be used. They supply the 6 tastes and also balance the energetics for each metabolic profile. They are called *churnas*. Vata churna is for people whose experience is of being cold, dry, "windy" and ungrounded, Pitta churna is for people who run "fiery" hot and impatient and Kapha churna is for people who find themselves and their digestion "watery" slow and heavy. Even if the "wrong" churna is used, it will not unbalance you.

The seasons of the year have an impact on our diet and lifestyle. It is always best to eat seasonally. Apples seem to be available year 'round but are only appropriate in the fall and however long they last in the root cellar during winter.

When the weather is dry and windy, it is better to avoid raw food and dry food. When the weather is hot, it is better to avoid hot, spicy or sour foods and becoming dehydrated. When the weather is cool and damp it is better to avoid cold, heavy mucus-producing foods. The seasons have an effect on diet and also on how we dress and in what activities we engage. For a person who runs hot, running in summer in the main part of the day is reserved for mad dogs and Englishmen.

Additional remedies in ayurveda include the use of humanized metals, gemstones, directional orientation and Vedic astrology (that describes when events will unfold rather than personality traits).

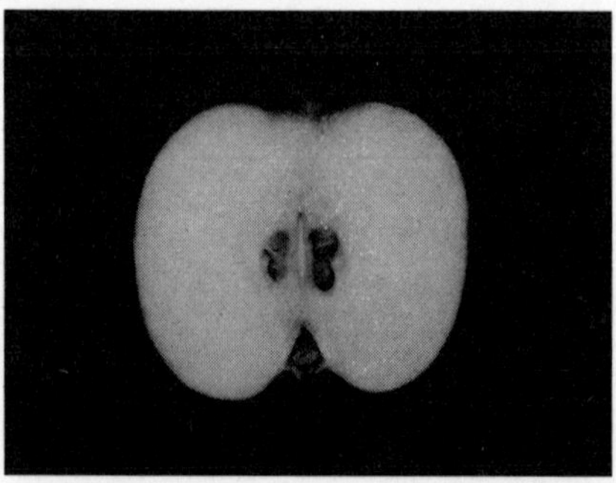

## Weeks 49 & 50 — FACIAL USING SPICES

Ayurveda teachings remind us that what we put on our skin is absorbed into the bloodstream and cells. It is very easy to work with homemade ayurvedic cosmetics as they are foods and spices and do not have to include chemical preservatives.

Skin-temperature or warmed cold-pressed oils are the best emollients and we use them for abhyanga and general oleation. Rose hip oil on the face is lovely and a small amount of evening primrose seed oil is as well. These will probably have preservatives but let's not stress over little bits. Everything we put on or in our body has an effect so just don't overdose.

For exfoliation and toning of the skin try the following recipe.

Mix together equal amounts of the ground powders of coriander, cumin, licorice and chickpeas (besan). Add a lesser amount of fenugreek powder. Whatever is not used can be stored in an airtight container for a few months.

Combine one teaspoon of the dry mix with warm milk if your skin is dry, warm water with a few drops of lemon juice if your skin is oily or warm water as is. The consistency would be thin enough to flow and thick enough to stick. Apply and massage your face and neck. Feel free to continue into body painting. Leave on a short time without it drying. If you engage someone in conversation, don't expect to be taken seriously. Rinse off first with warm water and then with cool. Complete with a pat of rose water if you wish (soak fresh rose petals in water in the sun for awhile) and a light application of abhyanga oil as is necessary. Do not exfoliate too often.

Other blends include turmeric and manjishta (*Rubia cordifolia*) that are good for the skin, and sandalwood, which is cooling.

The skin reflects our internal environment. If there are dark areas around the eyes, the salt and water in the body are not in proper relationship: you are using too much salt or not drinking enough water. Or you are not having enough exercise and the lymphatic system is sluggish. Or the bowel is not working well. If the eyes, mouth and tongue are puffy, your digestion is not working well. If there is acne, the body is throwing the toxins to the surface for elimination. Look at diet, lifestyle and perhaps include more bowel cleanses. If your skin is dry, look to the amount of oil in the diet and perhaps increase abhyanga.

## Weeks 51 & 52 — RETREAT WEEKEND

To celebrate a year of ayurvedic adventure, plan a retreat weekend. A weekend is one day longer than the typical bowel cleanse practice so you can luxuriate in time, doing all the good things you can for your body, senses, mind, heart and soul. You will further come to know that when you take care of yourself you are better able to take care of everyone and everything else.

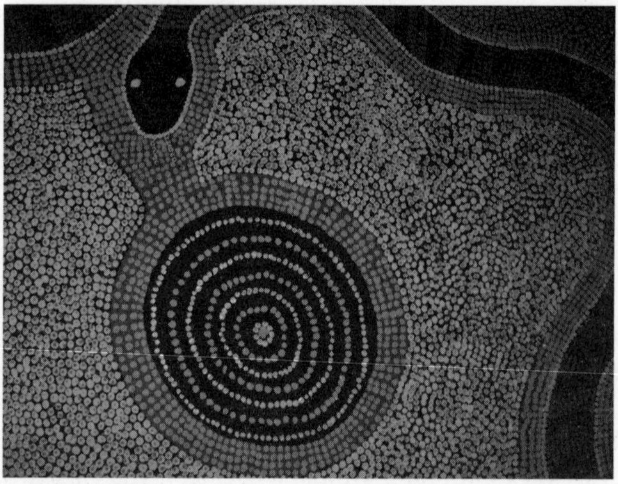

We all have responsibilities and commitments. It is good to get away by yourself or with friends once a year and rather than partying, shopping, engaging in sports and sightseeing, do a practice like this. Even though you will not be doing your usual home and work routine there will be plenty to do.

There are several options for this weekend in relation to bowel cleansing. You can prepare by softening and loosening ama as for the bowel cleanse in weeks 37 and 38. Or you can choose to start on Friday night with a bowel cleanse without previous preparation. Of you can leave out the bowel cleanse altogether.

What follows is a possible timetable for the weekend.

### FRIDAY EVENING

**6:00 PM**: Eat a light meal. Sit for five minutes after eating, then rinse your mouth and take a walk. Remember to follow these post-dining instructions for all meals.

**7:00 PM**: Read or listen to inspirational texts, chants or music or engage in pleasant conversation. If you are in the company of friends for the weekend, make an agreement amongst yourselves to steer away from flammable topics and heart-wrenching stories. This will take great awareness by each person. We are used to discussing our problems with people we feel comfortable with. And yet these problems are not actually occurring now. Make this a break from the outside world.

**8:30 PM**: Warm your massage oil and massage space and perform abhyanga if you have not done so today. Include a few drops of essential oil in your massage oil if desired. Play music if desired.

**9:15 PM**: Shower or bathe if you have done abhyanga or if desired. Get ready for bed with oral hygiene.

**10:00 PM**: Take the purgative if you are going to. Good night.

## SATURDAY

**6:00 AM**: Morning ablutions including toilet and oral hygiene.

**6:15 AM**: Hot water.

**6:30 AM**: Abhyanga in a warm space with warm oil, essential oils and music as you wish if you are not purging.

**7:00 AM**: Shower or bathe. Afterwards dress in clean natural fiber clothes for yoga.

**7:30 AM**: Yoga, breathing practice, relaxation, meditation and chanting.

**8:30 AM**: Complete your yoga practice.

If you are engaged in bowel purging you may feel like fasting until an early lunch. Or enjoy a cooked breakfast when hungry.

**The rest of the morning**: Circulate your activities amongst the following: Sit or walk in nature, read philosophical or inspirational texts, ponder spiritual art, listen to chanting or other agreeable music, chant, hum, sing to yourself and with the group, do another short yoga practice or lie in semi supine, listen and follow a guided relaxation, meditation or breathing practice, paint, draw, journal, write poetry, drink hot water, laugh, giggle, smile.

**Noon**: Enjoy a light lunch when hungry, the best choice being kichuri and ama-reducing broth or something similar. Perform post-dining actions.

**The afternoon**: Continue to rest and circulate your activities as in the morning. Afternoon rest can include a quarter to half hour nap but not just after eating. If you wish to nap, tell your mind to wake after 30 minutes, visualize that time on a clock. Tell yourself you will wake feeling alert and fine. We don't want to sleep all afternoon as that will impact on natural night sleeping.

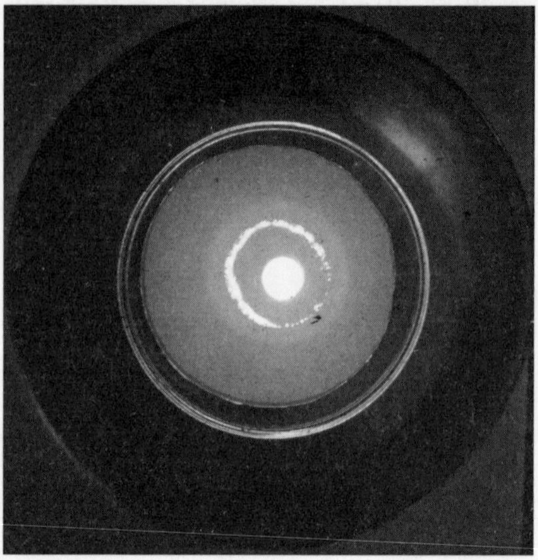

**4:00 PM**: Give yourself a facial and perform a late afternoon self-massage if you haven't enjoyed one in the morning.

**5:00 PM**: Shower or bathe.

**5:30 PM**: Everyone: repeat a yoga, breathing, meditation and chanting practice unless you have done several today already.

**6:00 PM**: Have your evening meal when hungry and include your post-dining practices.

**7:30 PM**: Trade with a friend or give yourself a head massage. Put on a beanie or scarf.

**8:30 PM**: Begin voluntary silence and retire early, no later than 10 PM. Sleep well, visionary dreams.

## SUNDAY

Repeat the routine presented Saturday. We are deepening our beneficial habits.

Practice noble silence if you are in a group until (at least) after breakfast. Notice where and why you want to talk. The sooner the ego gives up the need to express with language, the more energy we will seat in ourselves. Write in your journal if that helps. Notice if you become positively habituated to the mental rest that silence provides. Extending your exhalation can help quiet the need to speak. If you have been by yourself this weekend I trust you have had experience of simplicity and contentment, an inner silence and softness, which when radiating out causes everything to be experienced as peaceful and radiant.

Stay present in the time this weekend has given you as you have it, why rush it away?

As you prepare to leave the retreat, I believe you will feel refreshed and rejuvenated. Commemorate the changes that have occurred with a ritual that is representative to yourself or your group: a circle of self-expression, of chant, connecting with a token of nature, looking at some of your art or poetry....

Go outward, still centered in your own felt presence, a blessing to yourself and others.

A retreat is a good idea at the change of seasons so that we release the excesses of the former and have a more ama-free body and mind for come what may.

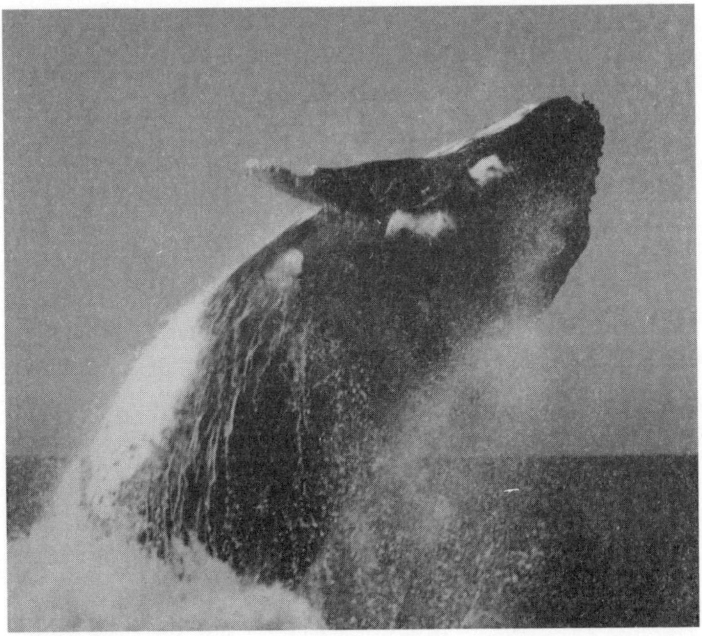

Additional recipes to enjoy on a retreat weekend or any time:

## JOB'S TEARS

Lachryma jobi is the Traditional Chinese Medicine grain of choice to promote good digestion.

Per person soak ¼-cup for 6-8 hours. Rinse and add water above the level of the grain. Bring to boil, lower heat and cook covered for 90 minutes. Keep topping up with water if necessary. In the last half hour add several chopped Chinese dates, a sprinkle of ginger, cinnamon and/or cardamom powder, a sprinkle of salt and one teaspoon of your choice of oil: ghee (clarified butter), coconut oil, almond oil or other nut oil. To make this savory instead of sweet, add Braggs Liquid Aminos, grated fresh ginger and one teaspoon from the above oil selection in the last quarter hour.

## FENNEL-CORIANDER TEA

Dry roast ¼-teaspoon each per cup. Remove to mortar when first seeds pop. Add water to the pot and bring to boil. Grind seeds coarsely and add to the water. Steep until drinking temperature. Both fennel and coriander help digestion without increasing heat.

## MUNG VEGETABLE SOUP

For three serves, wash ½-cup split mung beans. Soak if possible. Add 4 cups water, bring to boil, skim, cover and simmer. Stir at 20 minutes, adding 1 cup chopped zucchini or asparagus, 1 cup chopped broccoli or cabbage, ¼ cup chopped carrot or beetroot. Dissolve 1-teaspoon ghee on top of the soup; add ½-teaspoon fennel seed, 1-2 teaspoons of ground coriander and a pinch of asafoetida. Cover and continue cooking 5 minutes more. Stir; add rock salt or Braggs Liquid (sometimes called) Amigos to taste. Garnish with fresh coriander or basil.

## CHAPATI-S

Per chapati, combine ½-cup atta flour (soft wheat wholemeal, coarser bran sifted out), a sprinkle of rock salt, a sprinkle of cumin seed, ¼-teaspoon ghee and 1/6-cup water. (One-third liquid per amount of flour.) Knead into dough and let rest covered with damp cloth for 30-60 minutes if possible. Warm a heavy skillet or chapati pan over medium high heat. Roll out the dough and place on unoiled skillet. Adjust heat to prevent burning and cook until light brown on bottom. Flip and cook other side. If they puff up that's a good sign. Remove from pan and spread some ghee on top if desired. Serve warm---nothing like fresh warm chapati-s!

# Sanskrit Terms

**Abhyanga**
Massage with warm oil

**Ama**
Incompletely digested material from the physical, emotional and mental diets which remains lodged in the system and interferes with its proper functioning

**Ayurveda**
The holistic science of life and longevity

**Chapati**
A soft wheat unyeasted flatbread

**Churna**
"Powder", in this case spice blend powders

**Dosha**
The manifesting intelligence of the 5 great elements, ether, air, fire, water, earth, expressed in the body in certain combinations. See vata, pitta and kapha.

**Gandush**
The swishing of liquid or oil in the mouth to remove ama

**Jathara Agni**
"stomach fire"; the digestive enzymes and chemicals that break down food

**Kapha**
A genetic constitution that displays the qualities of earth and water; the dosha orchestrating cohesion, accumulation and lubrication in the body

**Kichuri**
Cooked split mung beans and rice with digestive spices

**Pitta**
A genetic constitution that displays predominantly the quality of fire with some water; the dosha orchestrating transformation in the body

**Prakruti**
Your natural genetic constitution incorporating all the dosha-s in your unique personal profile

**Sattwa**
The state of mind in which you are connected to the divine directive intelligence, thus promoting positive growth and fulfilment

**Vata**
A genetic constitution that displays the qualities of ether and air; the dosha orchestrating movement, communication and transport in the body

**Vikruti**
A state of imbalance in a person

**Yoga**
Union; the practice of energy-enhancing actions; a goal and the movement towards the goal

Totem

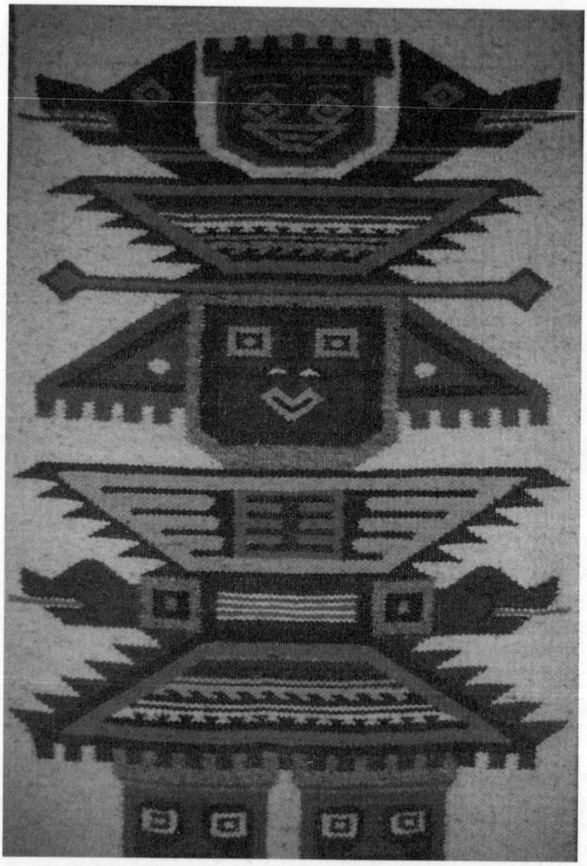

Tapestry, South America

# PRACTICE LOGS

Logs provide a record of how things went for you.
Create them with pens, crayons, paints on paper or design something on the computer.

## BOWEL CLEANSE LOG

Date

Purgative & quantity taken

Transit time

Duration

Comments

Transit time is how long it took the purgative to work from ingestion of the purgative to the first bowel movement. Duration is how many hours the emptying of the bowel continued.

## AMA-REDUCING DIET LOG

Day and date begun

Ama-reducing broth twice per day

Hot water three times per day unless you run hot, then let it cool somewhat

Hot ginger water three times per day after meals unless you run hot, then use roasted fennel seeds or mint

Aloe vera juice (certified by the aloe council) before meals

## ORAL HYGIENE LOG

Tongue and gandush daily

## ABHYANGA LOG

Full body two to three times per week in the next 7-14 days, unless you feel congested, in which case your body has absorbed sufficient oil and you can pause this until you feel uncongested, about 1-2 weeks

Head massage twice a week for two weeks

Ongoing body one to seven times a week

Ongoing head once or twice a week

## MEDITATION LOG

Daily practice ideally the same time each day

Morning

Evening

## EXERCISE LOG

Walking daily, weather permitting, average pace

Yoga or tai chi, chi gung, etc. Daily or at least three times a week

## PERSONAL NOTES

# PART TWO

## Expanding Understanding

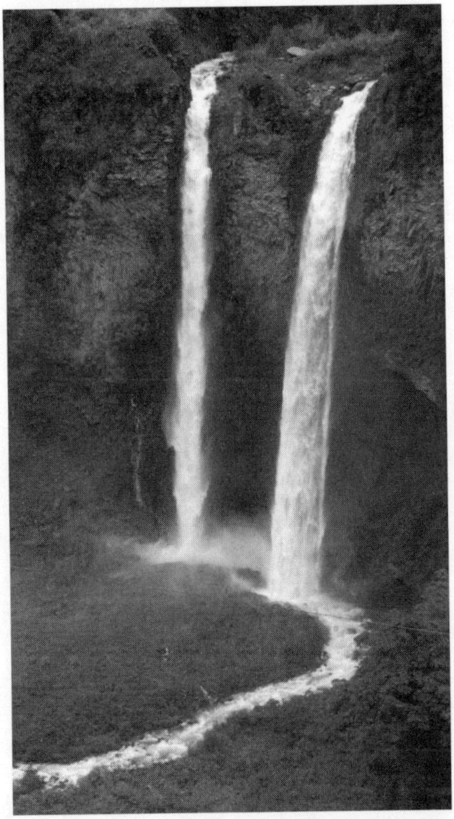

BY THIS TIME YOU ARE LIVING THE RECOMMENDATIONS of ayurveda because they work. Already standing on sacred ground, the clearer we are, the more we get it! You may have found that you respond best through your intellect supporting the why of the recommendations. Or through your actions supporting the how of them. Or through your feelings supporting your faith in them. We all need to soften and relax in order to heal.

You may wish to gain a broader appreciation of the concepts so that you can understand the recommendations of Part One, or when you consult with your ayurvedic practitioner or to determine your own requirements and remedies.

Allow what follows to live and breathe within you. Ponder the ideas, go out in nature and observe her signatures, look at the whole picture. Discuss it with health care consultants and friends, nurture your intuition and appreciate there are always exceptions to a rule, that at times concepts must yield. Whenever this information is re-read it will make more sense. Suddenly we see examples of what the teachings are referring to. This world offers, without its own agenda, myriad ways of relating to it.

Sanskrit, the language of ayurveda, is both grammatically complex and holistically poetic. Any Sanskrit word is a combination of sounds and signifies an idea on levels of experience from physical to spiritual. It causes the mind to integrate these levels and not define things so stringently. Allow this to be easy. It is an enlightening, ongoing process. When you connect with the wisdom of ayurveda you connect with wisdom at its source.

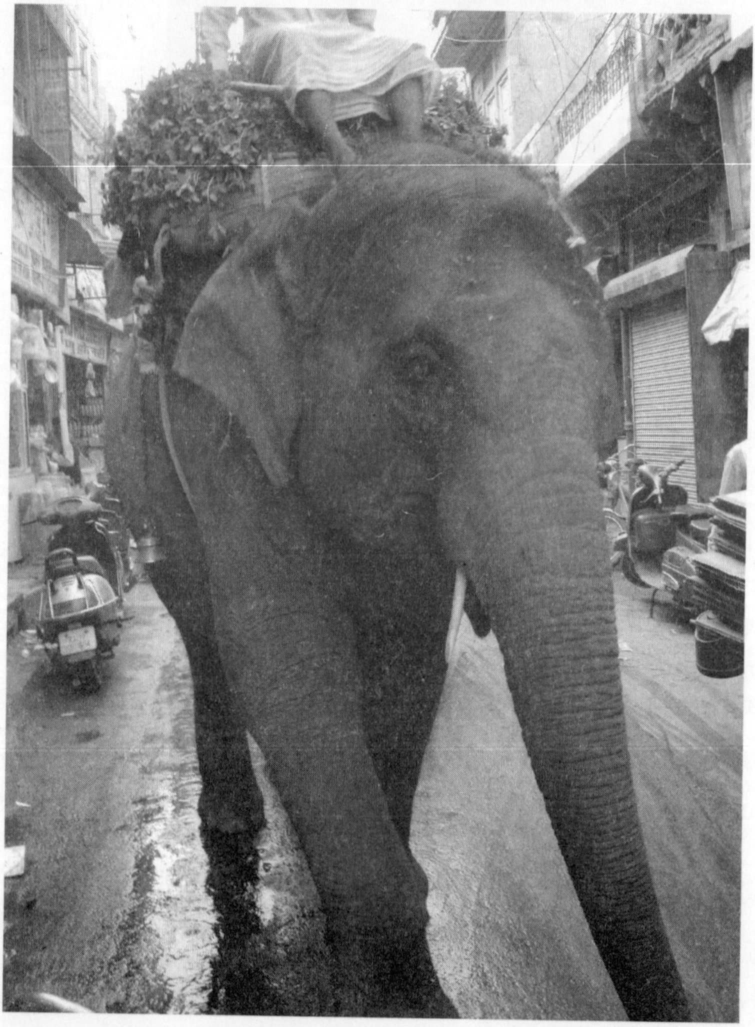

# THE SEVEN BASIC CONCEPTS

The World Health Organization regards ayurveda as "the world's most ancient, scientific, holistic, complete, natural system of healthcare". Originating in the Vedic wisdom from the mainland of India, it is based on principles that are as old as life itself.

### 1. The Unchanging Nature of Ayurveda

The basic principles have not changed because they are grounded in the laws of nature, which provide an expansive, stable foundation. Compare this with modern discoveries, which seem to come and go quickly and are only pieces of the whole.

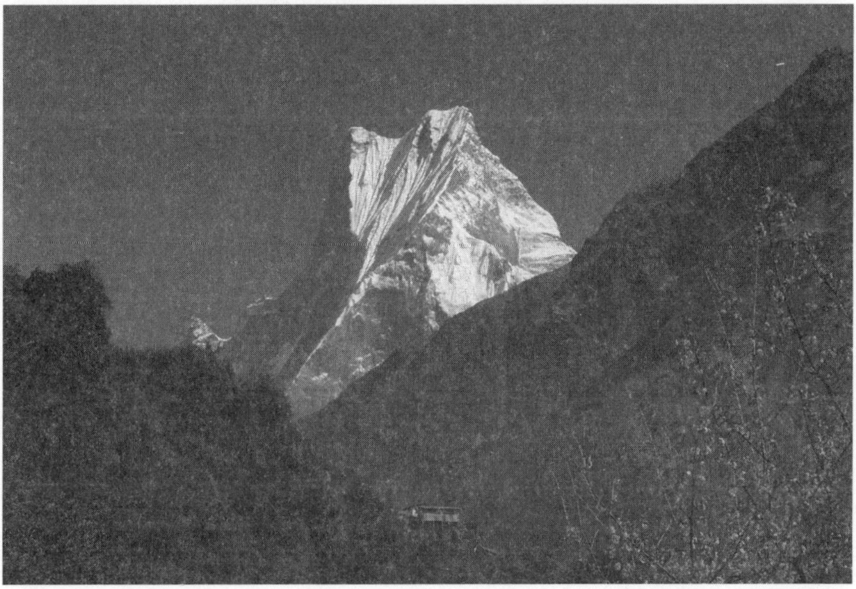

### 2. Subjectivity

Ayurveda has always included "gut feelings", inner knowing and intuition as part of its approach. The unseen intelligence cannot be pinned down by technology and life does not proceed from external verification of experience.

### 3. The Five Elements - Pancha Mahabhuta-s

The governing principles that give rise to and guide ether, air, fire, water and earth also operate within us because we are part of nature.

### 4. The Three Dosha-s

The pancha mahabhuta-s that comprise nature combine into three dosha-s to control all processes in human physiology.

VATA controls movement, drying and separation.

PITTA controls transformation.

KAPHA controls cohesion, growth and liquefaction.

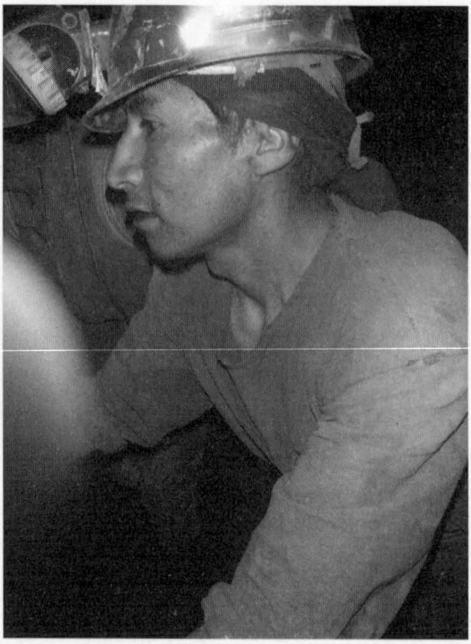

### 5. Prakruti

Your uniquely individual doshic profile present from birth brings its own ayurvedic instruction manual on how you can achieve balance in your life. Prakruti is one's true state.

### 6. The Effect of the Seasons

We live and interact with our environment that includes the movement of time as the seasons, the rhythms of sun, moon and earth, and varying proportions of air, fire and water. Ignoring the impact of heat and cold, of dry and wet, of still and windy, ignoring the impact of the seasons on us is the third cause of disease.

### 7. Panchakarma

The "five actions" provide ways to rejuvenate the body by purifying it of degenerating influences. When the blocks to our directive intelligence are removed, health flows freely.

# THE FOUR ASPECTS OF LIFE

The word *ayus* or life is defined as the inborn, intelligent co-ordination of our soul, mind, senses and body. It encompasses the sensation of life in us as us and the two-way interaction of our place in the world and the world's influence on us.

**Atma: The Soul**

In terms of embodied life this is the inner intelligence connected to universal intelligence, directing all aspects and providing dynamic equilibrium. The functioning and healing of the body is well beyond our capacity, both in understanding and coordination. That we breathe most of the time without thinking is atma at work through our respiratory system. Atma is always promoting harmony and health; it is part of the eternal supreme transmission of grace.

**Manas: The Mind**

This is the interpretative mechanism of human life. What we receive through our senses gets a "coloring" based on our past experiences. As an example, one person may hate thunderstorms, another love them. The storm does what it does and the mind colors the picture. There are many ideas that have become impressed on the subtle substance of mind and they dictate how we live, act and react. We would like experience to speak to us without the mind projecting these biases.

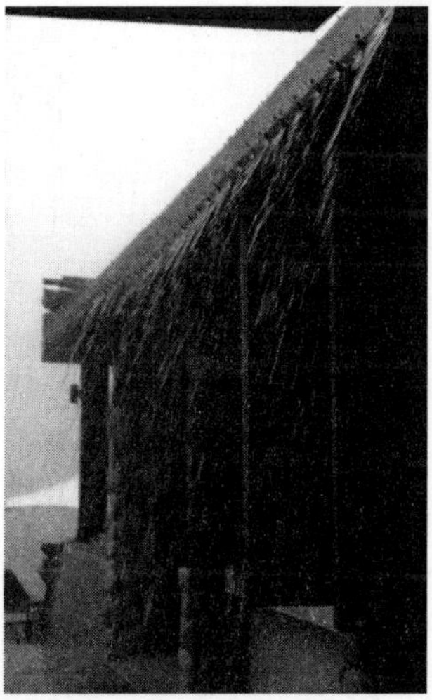

Ayurveda encourages re-education so that we operate from choice rather than habit. It also encourages awareness. The mind is *the* pivotal layer in our experience as humans and when we understand its functioning we are able to use it to promote a sane, serene, creative life.

**Indriya: The Senses**

We gather information about the environment and ourselves through our senses. Imbalances can arise due to insufficient sensory stimulation as well as bombardment. We can provide quality sensory input by choice, which then supports the mind-body. We can use our senses as part of the feedback process to decide if what we are doing is good for us. If your ears are ringing after listening to any genre of music, it was too loud. Misuse of the senses, asatmya-indriyartha-samyoga, is considered the second cause of disease because when we lose the protective function of our sense-ability, we rattle the mind and so make poor choices in terms of our wellness. The fast visuals in modern TV, film, etc. are one of the ways we rattle our minds.

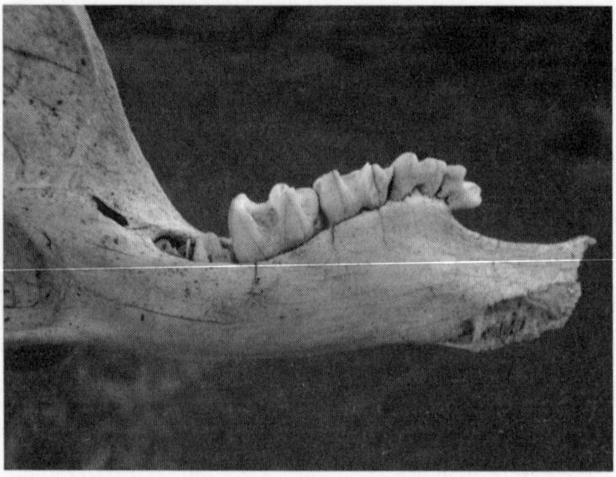

**Sharira: The Body**

Sharira is the most solid part of our existence and an innocent bystander to our uninformed or biased choices. Sharira represents ¼ of our total life experience. The body changes slowly compared to the mind, which is good in that we can experience where our minds have been. It's not so good because imbalance takes longer to undo at the physical level. Any restoration of health must address the non-physical domain, atma, manas and indriya. Through sharira we can influence manas and indriya in a positive way and integrate them with each other and atma. Examples of this are the diet and lifestyles we feed the body.

Imbalance can arise at any level and affect any level. When looking at imbalance look at your entire life: prakruti, diet, relationships, lifestyle, use of the senses, thoughts, environment. Each person's imbalance will have different factors entering and influencing it. Therefore, the same remedy, even for the same imbalance, will never be mindlessly suggested. A friend in all good faith may encourage us to use a remedy that worked for them but may not necessarily work for us.

# THE PANCHA MAHABHUTA-S

**Akasha: the principle of space**

The primary manifestation is the matrix. It is non-resistant, non-judgmental and allows everything. The sense of hearing is associated with it.

**Vayu: the principle of movement**

This governs all motion in the universe. Motion implies direction and causes drying and separation. The sense of touch is associated with it.

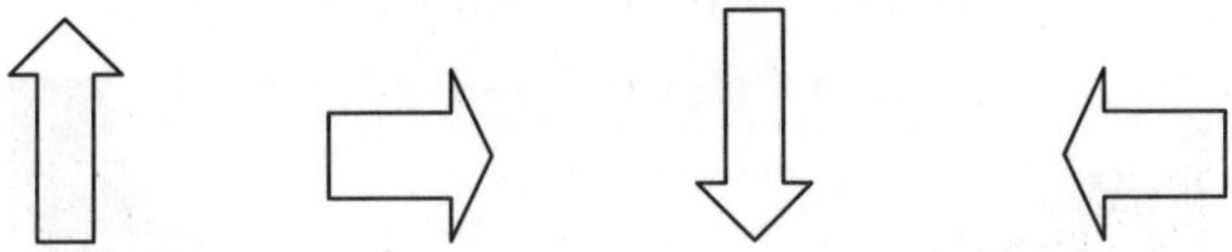

**Agni: the principle of conversion, heat and light**

As matter becomes denser, transformation and change can manifest. The sense of sight is associated with it.

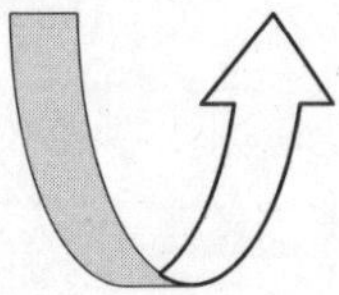

**Jala: the principle of cohesion and liquidity**

At this point matter starts to stick together and move without losing integrity. The sense of taste is associated with it.

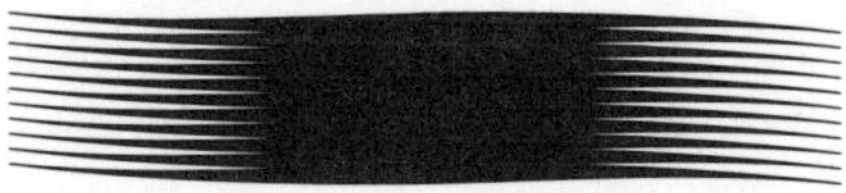

**Prithivi: the principle of form and structure**

That any particle exists is due to this principle. It is the least reactive of physical states, the densest and the last to manifest. The sense of smell is associated with it.

# PRAGYA APARADHA

**This is regarded as the primary cause of disease.**

It is the state where we think we are a physical entity having a spiritual experience when actually we are a spiritual being having a physical experience. This is the mistake of the intellect and puts us in a state of unconscious discord. We dwell excessively on the material plane. Reconsider that atma is the source of healing, not anything we can think up or manufacture. We support the healing process by affirming and experiencing that there is intelligence at work on our behalf. If there wasn't, we would still have every cut and bruise from childhood. If it works on the skin level, why wouldn't it work on the internal level or the mental level?

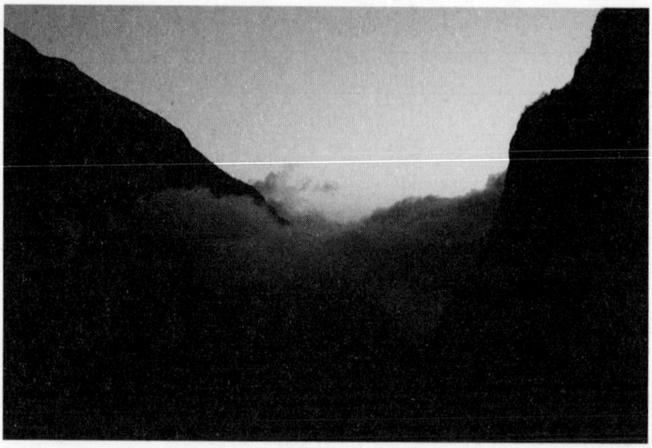

**What has happened to cause this spiritual amnesia, this veil over knowingness?**

Just as we trusted unconsciously that we would heal as a child, just as we learned to walk through all the falls we took, at that time the thinking, judging mind was immature. If thinking preceded walking we would all be immobile for the self-consciousness of falling so many times. It was when manas began to 'think' about life as it was presented, when the sense of self and environment were acquired, certain biases were built in. These have persisted without the discriminating aspect of buddhi re-evaluating them. The outer world is real and entertaining and over time causes manas to look for all solutions outwardly.

Mind in its more expansive definition functions in different modes. It synthesizes our impressions of the external world into a coherent experience, gives us a sense of identity, provides memory, discriminates what promotes wellness from what compromises it, accesses wisdom from a broader source and reflects physical experiences to atma.

This internal instrument is a non-physical entity. Everyday parts of it are affected by what we think, feel, sense, eat and drink.

We are aware of the placebo effect. If a person *thinks* a pill will lower his blood pressure, it can, even if it is a sugar pill.

**Emotions send certain chemicals through the blood, reaching every cell. Do you *feel* content or discontent?**

**What constitutes a beneficial *sensory* experience? What is the mind's bias to that experience? Are you having more good sensory experiences than disquieting ones?**

What we *eat and drink* can make us dull-witted, restless, or peaceful and satisfied.

Pragya aparadha can also mean crime against nature and wilful perversity. It indicates that we do things that are not in our best interests, knowingly or unknowingly. This happens because of our past mental conditioning or perhaps we have incorrect information or maybe we are just plain stubborn.

There is a simple explanation of this: the process of habituation is an evolutionary advantage yet it can take over our lives. If we had to re-learn everything everyday how could we flee predators? This same function causes us to do the same things over and over. It takes an effort of will over time to instil new desired habits. So act wilful with a purpose.

**How do we live in the solution to pragya aparadha?**

We are already doing so by following Part One recommendations. Diet, lifestyle, abhyanga, yoga, meditation and selfless service all contribute. The most direct method is daily meditation, where we come to examine manas. We compare the experience of agitated thinking with that of peace and contentment. We observe that the mind is like another person inside us (just the one, dear?) with an agenda of its own and that a percentage of its opinions are invalid or inappropriate. With this awareness we are able to put some time between the triggers that induce a certain reaction and the subsequent behavior. We can choose to think before reacting automatically. We can pause in the space and realize it's a past bias pushing us in a direction that we didn't choose. Delay the impulse even one second and have a symbolic word, gesture, giggle, which puts you at the point of choice, that makes the wave hover. Then re-route the impulse into a better form, something you have thought out already.

Simultaneously the feelings of universality, unity and harmony experienced during meditation open us to our true nature. Once the mind has relaxed, the same situation looks clearer. We experience ourselves as accepted and awesome and this helps healing. The veil begins to lift.

There are three states called guna-s that influence all of nature and manas moves between them. Guna is defined as attribute.

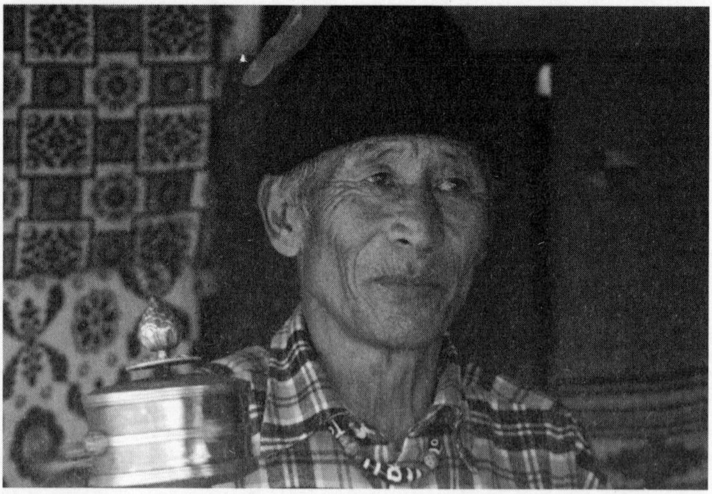

Sattwa guna is one of clarity, inspiration, balance, harmony and creativity. Both males and females have 70% mental sattwa. This is the mode that will benefit the planet and life on it, win-win, the greatest good for the greatest number. This is the shopkeeper who sells the customer a quality product and truly wants patrons to be satisfied. This is the philosophy known as utilitarianism.

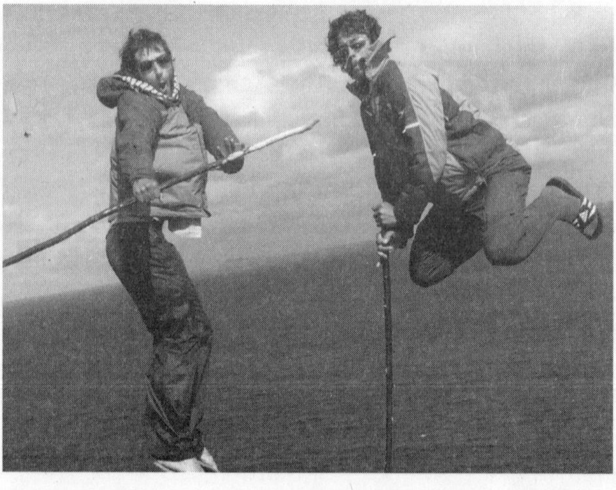

Rajas in the mind generates motivation, action and organization all of which we need to live in the world. Males have 20% rajas, females have 10%. Its dark side may be experienced as "I win, maybe you win if you support me, but I certainly win". There is also the feeling of existential hunger, wanting to devour everything.

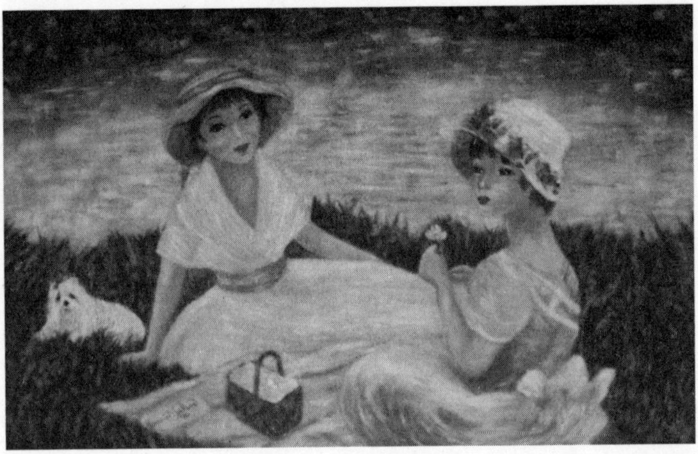

The mental state of tamas allows completion and rest. We want to turn off the light and be able to sleep at night. Females have 20% tamas, males have 10%. Its absolutely dark edge is "I win when you lose." As for a feeling, there is no feeling. From the inside there is no movement.

The sattwic mind always chooses things that are beneficial holistically, considering environment, others and oneself in measure. The mind becomes rajasic by hot, spicy, fried food, too many sweets, caffeinated beverages and excessive thinking or feeling. In this state one will stray from doing what is best for oneself and others and will feel driven to keep going and keep doing. The mind becomes tamasic, that is dull, heavy, inert, causing violence at times, by eating leftovers, fermented foods, too much red meat, drinking alcohol, taking drugs and becoming fatigued over a long period of time. In this state one will lose the plot altogether and the person may become destructive to self and others.

## Some Contributors and Indicators of Mental Constitution

| | SATTWA | RAJAS | TAMAS |
|---|---|---|---|
| DIET | Vegetarian | Some meat | Heavy meat diet |
| DRUGS, ALCOHOL | Never uses | Occasional use | Frequent use |
| SPEECH | Calm | Agitated | Dull |
| WORK | Selfless | Self-centered | Unmotivated |
| ANGER | Rare | Prone to | Frequent |
| DEPRESSION | Contented | Can oscillate | Deep depression |
| FORGIVENESS | With ease | With effort | Holds grudges |
| CONCENTRATION | Focused | Erratic | Distracted |
| VALUE SYSTEM | Important | Occasional | None |
| WILLPOWER | Strong | Variable | Weak |

# THE THREE DOSHA-S

The pancha mahabhuta-s begin as archetypes, as possibilities, as organising intelligences. They are not attached to anything. When they manifest it is in all of creation. When they interweave in our bodies we call them dosha-s. The dosha-s function in our psychophysical expression, bodily functions and in their essence are neither retained as tissues nor eliminated as natural wastes from the body. They do not start as a structure or a substance. They are formed in response to us having embodied life, causing our life processes to proceed and then would be spent. But dosha-s can accumulate and in excess affect the functioning and health of the body.

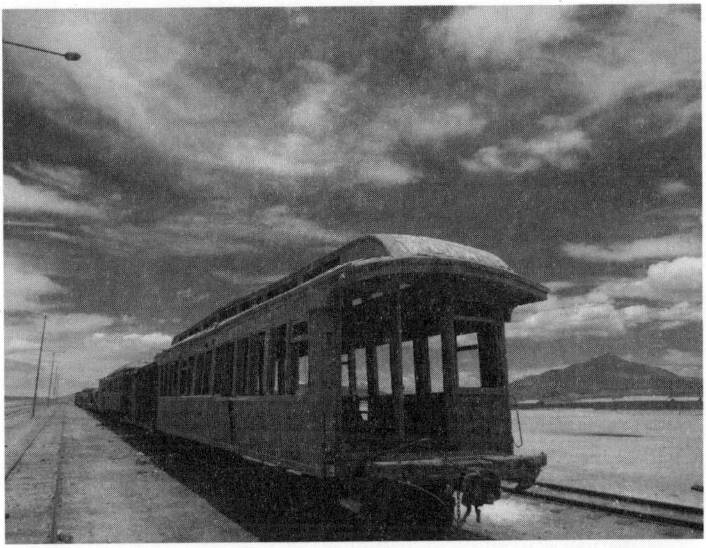

It is primarily akasha and vayu that join to become vata dosha so vata exhibits the qualities of ether and air. Ether is inert and exerts a lesser influence on us. The qualities of air are: dry, light, cold, rough, subtle and mobile. This results in absorbing, reducing, cooling, scraping, pervading and stimulating actions. Think of vata as air molecules expanding into ongoing space forever, voyagers in the universe. Think of vata as never holding on, not even to what is beneficial.

Pitta dosha is primarily agni, fire, then jala. Its qualities are: slightly oily, penetrative, hot, light, spreadable, liquefaction and sour smell. This results in adhering, penetrating, heating, reducing, spreading, liquefying and fermenting actions. I think of pitta as the intelligence that allows fire and water to live in our bodies without each trying to outdo the other.

It is primarily jala and prithivi that join to become kapha dosha so kapha exhibits the qualities of water and earth. Earth is considered slow to change in our bodies. Kapha qualities are: heavy, cold, soft, oily, sweet, steady and sticky. The actions are building, cooling, stabilizing, healing, moistening and adhering. Kapha can be mellow such as still water and sand not interacting or complacent in a major way like water and cement setting into concrete.

## MORE ABOUT DOSHA-S

Continue to create a profile of signatures of the dosha-s with the following information.

| | VATA | PITTA | KAPHA |
|---|---|---|---|
| COLOR | Black, purple | Red, yellow, green | White |
| LIFE STAGE | Middle age onwards | Puberty to middle age | Birth to puberty |
| WORSE IN | Cold, windy, dry | Hot, humid | Cold, wet, rainy, snowy |
| ACTIVE AT | 2-6 AM<br>2-6 PM | 10 AM-2 PM<br>10 PM-2 AM | 6-10 AM<br>6-10 PM |

## FUNCTIONS OF THE DOSHA-S

**VATA, the conductor**

- energy
- kindling digestion
- co-ordination of senses
- cardiac, nerve and muscle activity
- respiration, circulation and elimination
- movement of nutrients into cells and waste products out of cells
- all movement of and in the body
- homeostasis in the body
- equilibrium of tissues
- emotions

**PITTA, the transformer**

- courage
- heat regulation
- hormones and enzymes
- color of substances in body
- understanding, intelligence, mental perception, discrimination
- all digestion & conversion: mental, emotional, sensory, food
- complexion, lustre of skin and eyes
- visual perception
- hunger, thirst

**KAPHA, the builder and stabiliser**

- emotional calm
- cohesion, structure and stability
- lubrication of membranes, joints and wherever there is movement
- mental, emotional, physical, cardio-respiratory endurance
- forgiveness and compassion
- healing capacity
- taste

## ZONES AND LOCATIONS OF THE DOSHA-S

| KAPHA ZONE | KAPHA LOCATIONS |
| --- | --- |
| Upper 2/3 of stomach | Chest |
| Pericardium, heart | Trachea, vocal cords |
| Trachea, bronchi, lungs | Head, brain |
| Esophagus, pharynx, larynx | Palate/Tongue |
| Tongue | Stomach, Pancreas |
| Sinuses | Plasma |
| Middle ear membrane | Adipose tissue (fat) |
| Sense organs | Nose |
|  | Cerebrospinal fluid |
|  | Synovial joint fluid |

Kapha zone is associated with moistening, mixing together, binding and lubricating. Secretions are mainly white or pale.

| PITTA ZONE | PITTA LOCATIONS |
|---|---|
| Lower 1/3 of stomach | Intestines |
| Duodenum; ileum up to ileocecal valve | Lower 1/3 of stomach |
| Liver | Sweat glands |
| Spleen | Blood- red blood cells |
| Pancreas | Plasma |
| Gallbladder | Eyes |
| | Skin |
| | Brain |

Each of these organs produces substances containing acids or enzymes, which can be colored red, yellow or green. These substances produce transformation.

| VATA ZONE | VATA LOCATIONS |
|---|---|
| Colon | Colon/rectum |
| Bladder | Pelvis |
| Kidneys and ureters | Thighs |
| Uterus | Ears |
| Reproductive organs | Bones |
| Pelvic bones, hip joints, femurs | Skin |
| | Hair |

Space, dryness, lightness and movement are found here. Secretions are reabsorbed or held for elimination. The bones are larger. In the body, bones create spacious cavities for the brain and the organs.

Although the dosha-s have their domains, each is found in every cell throughout the body. They interact with each other. Each dosha is best suited to maintain health in its own locations because it has the specialised ability to nourish those tissues and to remove imbalances there. The dosha can distinguish between substances that are retained by the body and those that need to be eliminated. When ama blocks that intelligence, health is compromised.

Vata governs the other 2 dosha-s. When it is out of balance it can disrupt or block the others or move them to other locations. This is why ayurveda looks to pacifying vata as the first dosha and why the majority of diseases are vata derangements. Vata is linked to the physical body and the food that goes into it and vata is the pace at which we live, breathe and eat. By adopting good intake through food and a sane and serene life and mind, vata will be more balanced, thus supporting health.

The dosha-s work from the deepest tissues to the periphery, with vata bringing nourishment into body and wastes out of the body. Each dosha is active in its time period and is most efficient in its work and zone at that time.

**Agnidevaya Namaha**

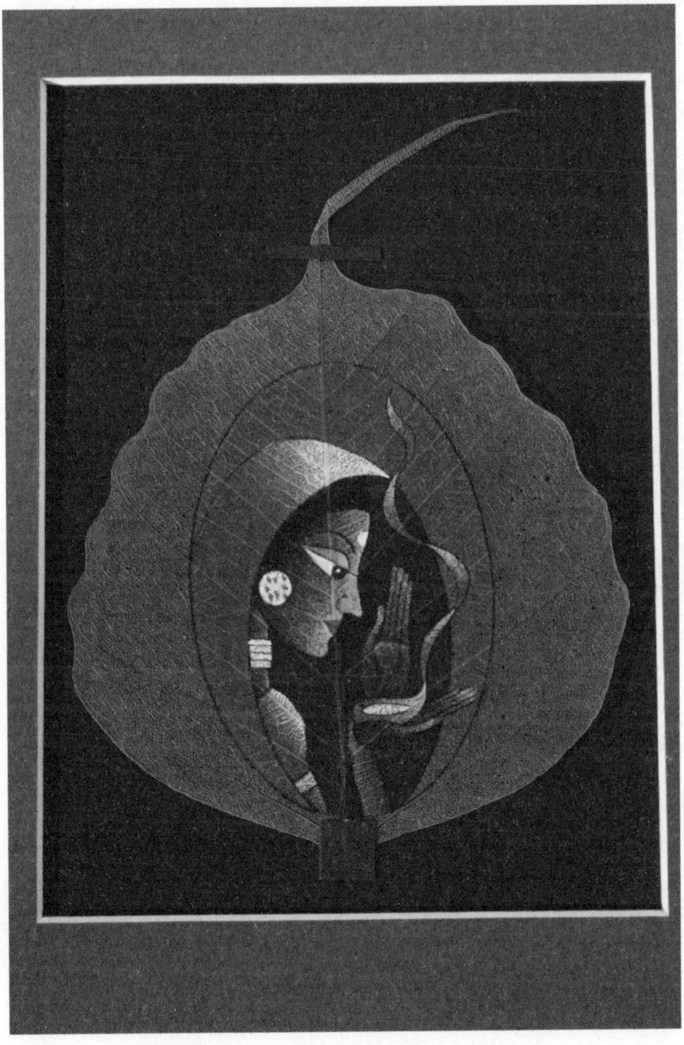

**paint on dried peepul leaf, India**

# PRAKRUTI and VIKRUTI

Nature plays the elements in us through our dosha-s like a musicologist's work at a sound mixer. We are a certain amount each of vata, pitta and kapha adding up to 100% and each of those dosha-s can be strongly expressed or not. Our basic tune has been laid down at birth. If we uphold it, the song is unique and clear. This is our state of prakruti. It has been influenced by the dosha-s in the sperm, semen and ovum, the quality and type of food eaten by mother, her lifestyle, the conditions within the uterus and the effect of the seasons on her during pregnancy. It means nature *and* our individual nature. A person can have one dosha in majority, or be bidoshic or tridoshic (rare).

## SOME INDICATORS FOR PRAKRUTI ARE:

VATA creative, variable, cold, dry

With the qualities of vayu, vata is lightweight. The body frame is thin and stamina is low. Features can be uneven or crooked. Vata people run cold and dry. Thoughts are creative, quick, inventive and flexible, movements are quick. Wind can shift easily and so can vata. From one day to the next appetite, digestion and interests can change.

PITTA intense, penetrating, sensitive, hot

This is the mesomorph body frame with more stamina that a larger system provides. With agni being predominant, coloring is more reddish, appetite and digestion are stronger; body heat, perspiration, odor and thirst are noticeable. Pitta intellect is witty and insightful and likes to manage people and ideas. Pitta is courageous and warm.

KAPHA heavy, cool, steady, moist

If vata is a little bird and pitta a little sun, kapha is a cushy little whale. The body frame can be wide/ deep/ tall. There is more bone, muscle, fat and larger organs, more structure, higher body mass index. Slow to get going, with more stamina, slower to learn with better long-term memory, slower digestion, kapha doesn't change quickly. Skin is cool and moist to the touch. Kapha energy holds on to everything and loves people, plants and animals.

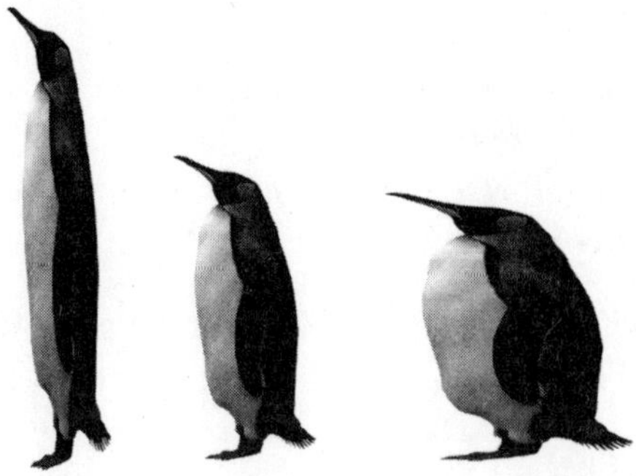

**Which silhouettes remind you of a vata person? Pitta? Kapha?**

Prakruti is already perfect in its individuality. We don't have to correct it. But we can unbalance it and that is a state called vikruti, meaning discordant with nature.

With the dosha profile classifications we play with in books or on the Internet, what we think is our prakruti may really be our vikruti because our innate propensities have been covered over by years of poor habits. There is sometimes a vata person under all those layers of adipose tissue. Ayurvedic physicians can come closer to knowing prakruti with pulse diagnosis but even this can be misleading if your pulse is unclear due to imbalance. We don't have to do anything about our prakruti but we do have to rebalance the vikruti. If vikruti deteriorates into chronic disease we may even change our prakruti.

When looking to correct an imbalance, your consultant will ascertain whether a dosha is blocked by ama or not. If blocked by ama the dosha has accumulated as a "spoiled" physical substance that obstructs the proper functioning of the body and needs to be removed. What has caused that? And are the dosha-s operating in excess or are they depleted? Are they in their proper locations or has vata moved them? We look for signs in the body, mind and behavior.

## VATA VIKRUTI

When vata is in excess there would be some or all of the following: coldness, dryness, excessive movement, nervous system instability, sensory malfunction and psychological difficulties. The person will seek warmth. There can be a purple/black tinge to the skin. Fear, worry and anxiety can worsen. Insomnia, fatigue and restlessness may be apparent.

In vata dosha depletion there can be exhaustion, less talking, less movement, sensory loss and insomnia.

## PITTA VIKRUTI

When pitta is in excess there would be some or all of the following: excessive heat, thirst and appetite, a yellow tinge to the skin and secretions, increased hot emotions like anger, resentment and criticism. Sleep is disturbed and there is a desire for cold things.

Depletion may show up as poor digestion and loss of appetite, pallor, insomnia and feeling cold.

## KAPHA VIKRUTI

When kapha is in excess there would be some or all of the following: heaviness, moistness, coldness and lethargy.

When depleted there may be dryness, a feeling of emptiness, giddiness, vertigo, palpitations, unstable or weak joints and burning in the upper stomach area.

Ayurveda attends to removing the cause of the problem, enhancing agni, reducing ama, balancing vata, then pitta, then kapha dosha. Much of the time we over-use our prakruti until it becomes a vikruti. Vata people may rush around too much or eat dry rough foods and drink astringent or bitter beverages without realizing that this will produce more vata symptoms. Pitta people may indulge their penchant for spicy foods and alcohol or continue to be very intense without realizing this will produce more pitta symptoms. Kapha people may settle back into inactivity or consume too many milk or wheat products without realizing that this increases kapha.

Yet all prakruti-s can experience all vikruti-s as well. For example, if we have a cold, no matter our prakruti, we have a kapha imbalance. The cause could have been leaving the house in the morning with wet hair, or working in an air-conditioned office, or eating cold dairy, or the change to winter season or even not enough rest, which can trigger any imbalance. Cold is an attribute of both vata and kapha. However a cold implies mucus, which is not an attribute of vata and is one of kapha. This mucus is excess kapha dosha and needs to be removed. To dry out a cold, avoid cold, moist food and environments. Eat warm, spicier foods that have a drying quality. Keep yourself warm and your head and upper body covered. Correct the factors that caused the imbalance. These guidelines are general because if we have a fever the body had produced warmth and we need to sweat. A vata cold may include a dry cough, a pitta cold may include green or yellow mucus.

Atma will do the job of rebalancing and we help by not suppressing the symptoms (which will only drive them deeper) or exacerbating them.

# THE SEVEN DHATU-S and MALA-S

Dhatu is that which is retained by the body and replenished or rejuvenated. It gives substance and strength. It may be thought of as tissue and it is also function. Excessive loss of any dhatu is unnatural and dangerous. The loss of reproductive tissue is natural. However, gentlemen, sexual continence is an advantage to your health. Mala is natural waste. Its elimination helps maintain body function. If retained, excessive or deficient, it can alert us to imbalance and needs correcting.

## THE SAPTA DHATU-S, THEIR FUNCTIONS AND MALA-S

| | | | |
|---|---|---|---|
| RASA | Plasma, Lymph | Nutritional fluid | Mucus |
| RAKTA | Red blood cells | Life support | Bile |
| MAMSA | Muscle | Movement | Ear wax, sebum |
| MEDA | Adipose (fat) | Lubrication | Sweat |
| ASTHI | Bone | Structure | Hair, nails |
| MAJJA | Marrow, Nerves | Communication | Unctuousness |
| SHUKRA | Sperm, Ova | Reproduction | None |

From shukra no secondary tissue or waste is produced but rather OJAS, the glow of health and immunity that circulates through the body, nourishing all dhatu-s.

Each dhatu is formed and nourished in the aforementioned sequential order with rasa formed from the available nourishing essence of the foods we eat.

The upadhatu are the secondary tissues.

From rasa is produced the outer layer of skin, breast milk and menstrual fluid.

From rakta is produced small tendons and blood vessels.

From mamsa is produced the 6 deeper layers of skin and subcutaneous fat.

From meda is produced flat muscle, tendons and ligaments.

From asthi is produced teeth and cartilage.

From majja lacrimal secretions (tears) are produced.

THE THREE MAJOR MALA-S ARE:

1. purisha-feces, the natural waste from food, eliminated via the colon
2. mutra-urine, the natural waste from metabolism and excess water, eliminated via the kidneys
3. sweda-sweat, the natural waste from adipose tissue, eliminated via the skin

Included in ayurvedic anatomy are myriad channels that convey, among other things, fluids, nerve impulses and consciousness.

It is the dosha-s that are responsible for the coordination of anabolism, metabolism and catabolism. Vata transports, pitta converts and kapha binds. Vata also dries. The dhatu-s have no overarching intelligence to decide if they should be retained. The mala-s do not decide to eliminate themselves. We appreciate how atma works in the physical dimension by understanding the relationship of dosha, dhatu and mala. Dosha is the inherent software that also becomes hardware to produce substances in the proper amount for the processes of life and guide dhatu-s that carry out their respective functions. These processes then naturally produce mala.

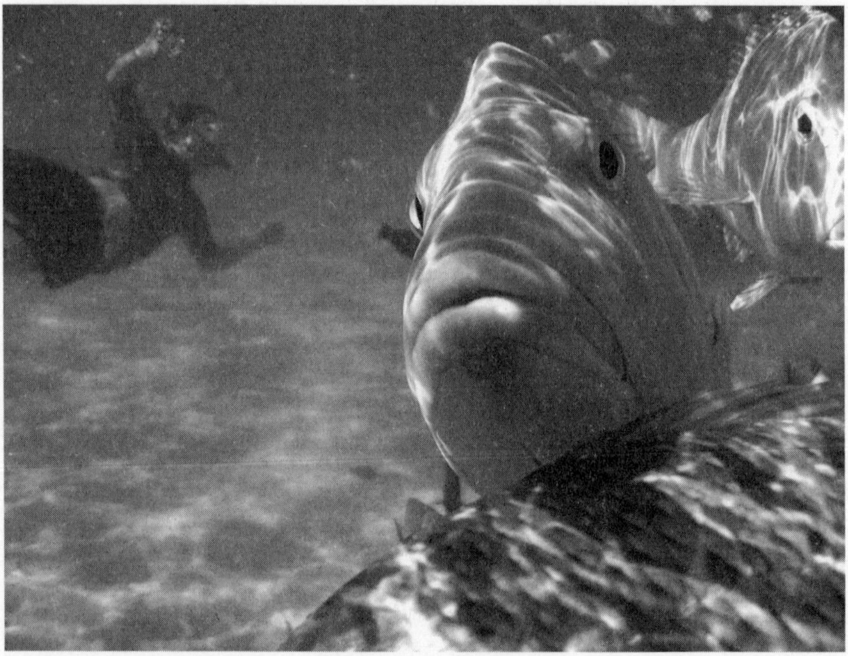

# THE SIX TASTES

Everything in nature is composed of and influenced by the mahabhuta-s. Through each sense we can balance or unbalance ourselves. Aromas, the texture of the clothes we wear, the color scheme of our living space, all support us or create an undefined sense of disquiet. With the sense of taste, each dosha is pacified by three tastes and aggravated by three others.

NOTICE WHICH MAHABHUTA-S COMPRISE EACH TASTE.

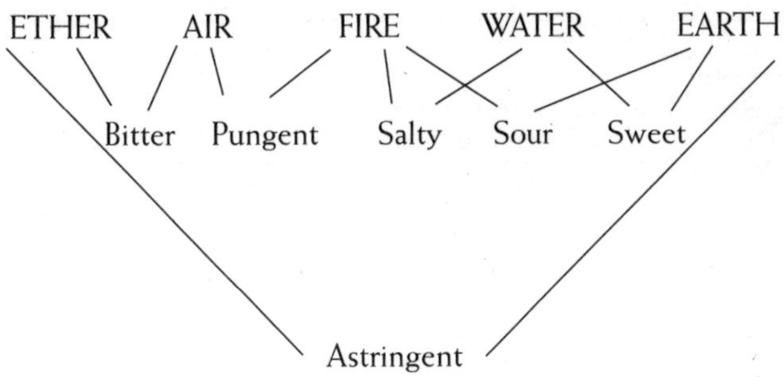


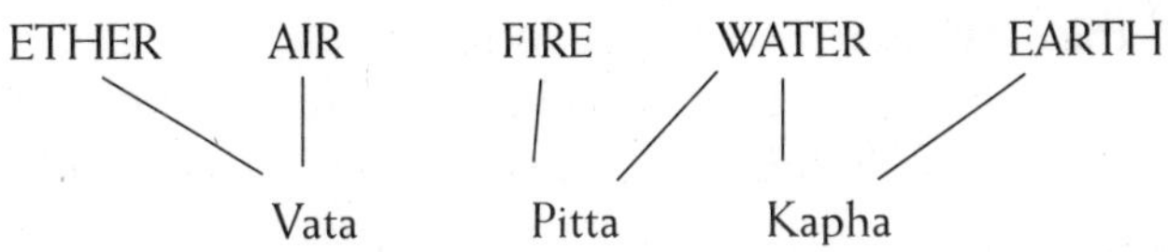


Vata is increased by bitter, pungent and astringent.

It is lessened by salty, sour and sweet.

Pitta is increased by pungent, salty and sour.

It is lessened by bitter, astringent and sweet.

Kapha is increased by salty, sour and sweet.

It is lessened by pungent, bitter and astringent.

## FILL IN THE BOXES GAME

Choose from the following attributes and find 3 that will increase each dosha and 3 that will decrease it. These qualities are referring to food but can describe other conditions.

Light Heavy Hot Cold Oily Dry

| Increases vata | Increases pitta | Increases kapha |
|---|---|---|
| | | |
| | | |
| | | |

| Decreases vata | Decreases pitta | Decreases kapha |
|---|---|---|
| | | |
| | | |
| | | |

## DESCRIPTION OF TASTES

Food with the salubrious sweet taste forms the majority of our diet. It is found in everything that grows. It builds our tissues and provides energy. Dietary sources are carbohydrate, protein, natural sugars and oils.

The salty taste is found in mineral salts and sea vegetables. Salt stimulates digestion, is a mild laxative and enhances all other tastes.

The sour taste as organic acids is found in citrus and other fruits and certain sour greens. This taste promotes appetite and digestion.

The pungent taste is found in pungent greens and ginger. The essential oils of herbs and spices such as oregano and black pepper also provide this taste. It helps stimulate digestion and dries congestion.

The bitter taste is detoxifying, anti-inflammatory and kindles the digestive fire. It is found in bitter greens, citrus rind, aloe vera, coffee, pure chocolate, and herbs and spices such as cumin and fenugreek. It is the taste of most pharmacopeia remedies.

The astringent feeling is what contracts the membranes of the mouth. Tea, dried beans, unripe fruit and herbs and spices with natural tannin can provide this drying, compacting action.

If all six tastes are present in a meal with attention to prakruti, vikruti and the season, we will receive proper nutrition and feel satiated. When we feel hungry after having eaten it can be because we have not included all the tastes in the meal. If we overdo a taste it also implies we are consuming too much of some elements, which will lead to imbalance. For example, a meal of predominantly pickled vegetables and cheese (sour, salty) is going to increase pitta. If pitta people have this in summer they are going to get even hotter and more impatient. A meal of lettuce on cracker washed down with a quick black iced tea (cold, dry, astringent) is going to increase vata. If vata people have this in cool, windy weather they are going to get even more dry, cold and unsettled. A meal of cold macaroni salad and ice cream (cold, sweet, heavy) is a kapha nightmare. If kapha people have it in winter or cool, rainy, snowy weather it will increase heaviness and congestion perhaps to the point of a cold or flu.

Use churna-s on foods, tempering them in ghee to make them more potent or use them to make a hot or warm spice drink.

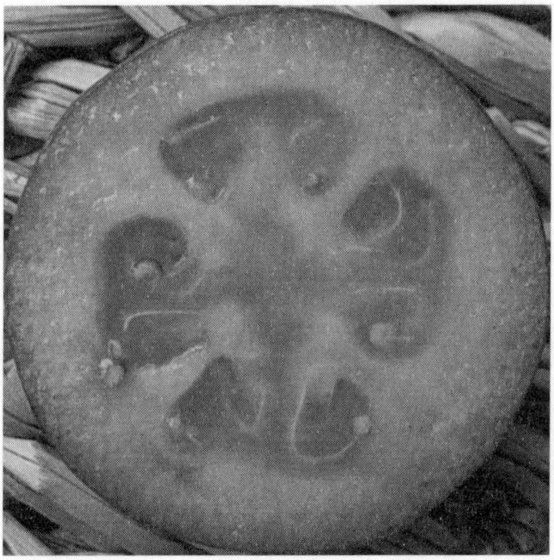

# PANCHAKARMA, THE FIVE ACTIONS

Unique to the teachings of ayurveda is the saving grace of these five actions. If we have ama deep in our tissues these procedures along with preparation and completion techniques can help expel it. This is as close as we can get to washing from the inside out.

Nasya treatment removes ama from the head and neck. Vamana removes it from the upper stomach and lungs. Virechana removes it from the lower stomach, small intestine, liver, gall bladder and pancreas. Raktamokshana removes it from the blood. Basti removes it from the colon and also replenishes the body through this site.

Panchakarma is its own branch of ayurveda and takes years of study and refined clinical application by the doctor. Southern India has a long history of panchakarma and many panchakarma centers. Read about Kerala panchakarma in Part Four.

Just as we do a mini-version by softening and loosening the ama prior to a bowel cleanse, the ayurvedic doctor does so with diet, massage, steam and other treatments, yoga and herbs. The minimum length of pre-treatment is about 7-10 days and that will provide only one grand clean-out, usually as virechana. It takes several to make a difference as each one goes in deeper, faster and brings out more ama. Post-treatment of 5-7 days is ideal so that we recuperate from this type of cellular microsurgery - removal of ama - and begin a rejuvenation process for the tissues.

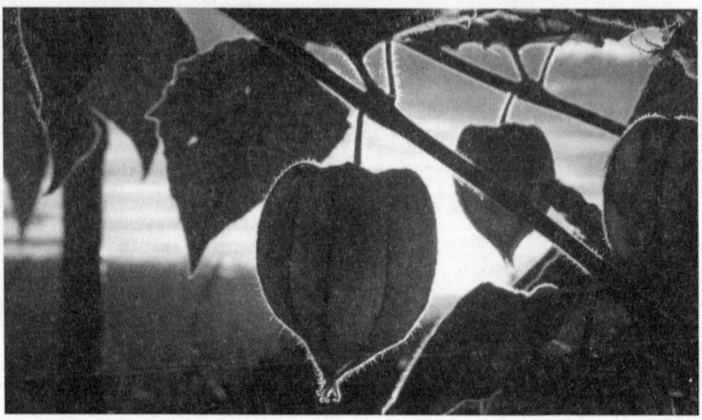

## WHAT'S ALL THIS FOR THEN?

Human consciousness is awareness itself. We can integrate information past, present, future, objective and subjective into a holistic understanding faster than the speed of thought. This is beyond the function of the brain and mind; it is the function of atma.

We have enumerated many aspects in Part Two because enumeration is one of the underlying philosophical schools of thought in India: how things arose, how many, and in what order.

The three pillars that support health are 1–what we take into our bodies through our senses, minds, breath, food, beverage and environment 2–how we use our energy in our day-to-day activities and 3–rebalancing when needed with diet, lifestyle, herbs and treatments. This last pillar also includes rejuvenating our rebalanced tissues.

Ayurveda reminds us to use our inner knowing, to look to the ways of nature, and to acknowledge that atma, manas, indriya and sharira influence each other to create an outcome. It teaches us that to stay balanced we become proactive in our choices with regard to lifestyle, diet, who we associate with, sensory experience and our own thoughts. It reminds us to accommodate climate and weather. It gives us guidelines on how to do so. We simplify back to the mahabhuta-s, the five elements, and assess how they are operating in and around us.

**What is the ayurvedic life exactly?** There are some useful things we eat and some useful things we do to start the ball rolling and the rest is our choice. Those choices become more aligned with what is beneficial for us as they reflect natural law. As we come to feel blessed, we are a blessing to everything we come into contact with.

We are all somewhat different from each other and different ourselves day to day. If we are new to these teachings or have become distanced from our own inner guidance, we can at any time begin to make changes. We start from where we are, right here, right now. Don't wait for the 'right moment' because the mind will come up with more excuses than you can imagine. That is pragya aparadha. Everyone engages in the same activity anyway, whether we are overweight, underweight or somewhere in between: to enhance our diet, lifestyle and mental disposition each day so as to enjoy this divine play.

In the flow, remembering that we are spiritual beings and honoring others and ourselves as such, yoga recommends that we take just one step and consolidate there. We want our sense of self to feel solid ground beneath our feet, to still recognize itself while we change slowly. Spend time with a new habit or understanding. From that vantage choose the next step. We don't know what that next step will be until we're looking from the new vista. This is one reason why it is unproductive to think too far ahead. It will get easier because as pragya aparadha clears, atma guides.

Becoming more in harmony with what and how we want to be means we are going in the right direction. If you find that living in the universe is immensely awesome, smile. Acknowledge with appreciation that when you feel awe, gratitude, divinity, flow, clarity, wellbeing, you are already within and always have been within the embrace of the Divine.

**Mumtaz Mahal**

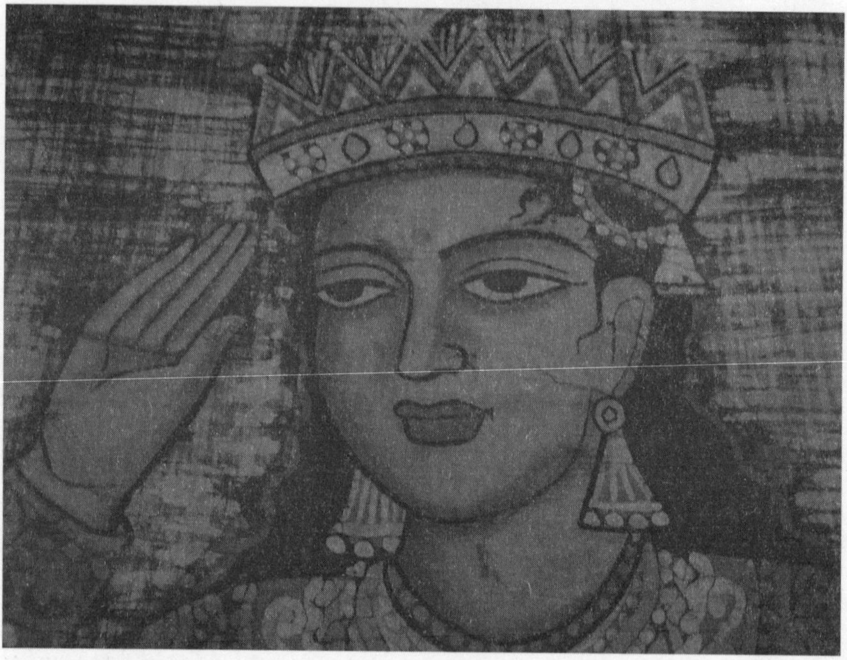

**Batik, India**

# Part Three

## Embellish The Recommendations

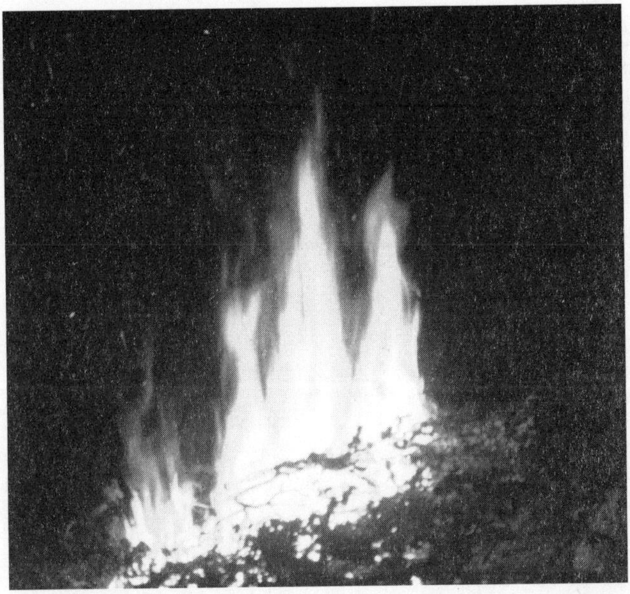

THE TEACHINGS OF AYURVEDA WORK WHEN WE USE THEM. Their gift is that they provide time-tested ways of maintaining health through intake and through lifestyle choices. The teachings also provide ways of clearing ama from the body-mind-heart before imbalance is compounded into disease. And they support our recognition of spirit in everything.

It is easier to stay well than to get well. The body can be in Stage Four of imbalance and we can still reverse it. Even with disease, Stages Five and Six, ayurveda gives us a better quality of life. And many pets have benefited from owners sharing their practices of ayurveda.

What has been entrained at an early age may seem to be tolerated, which is why we don't notice negative effects. If you find a recommendation is way out of line with your diet or lifestyle, please consider that a change will benefit you. For me it was bagel, cream cheese and lox. First the bagel went, I found it was always heavy to digest, even toasted. Then I read that mixing fish with dairy creates digestive commotion. (See FOOD WISDOM below.) Then I chose not to consume the more sentient beings. I'm not pining for the old food: been there, eaten that, moving on.

Wellness is not limited by age or gender; it can be limited by resistance, misinformation and sleeping while awake.

We all lapse now and then so begin again and again with ayurveda. You'll slip into the recommendations with greater ease each time.

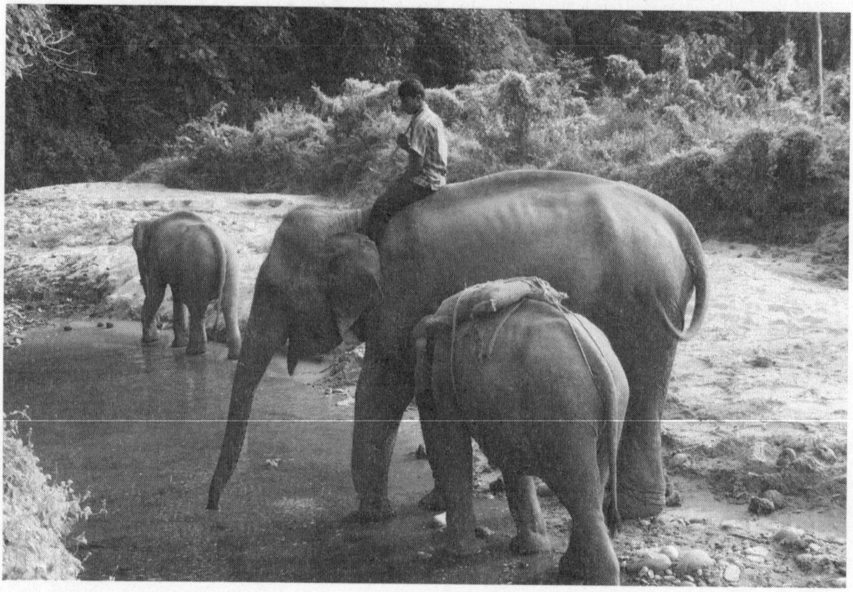

# THE AYURVEDIC DAY

There are practices that align us to the natural energies of day and night and the rhythms of nature. Have appreciation for the following sequence, considering why we would do this action at this time rather than at another time. You might not do all the morning recommendations each morning. Allot some personal time and do one, rotating through them through the week. Although the following progression is regarded as harmonious there is also allowance for individual needs. If you get hungry before you reach that recommendation, please eat. That is a primary urge that should not be postponed. Include yoga in action, making breakfast, lunch and dinner for your family. To do so with love is part of the ayurvedic day, with the other recommendations making space for it. Doing some housework or gardening prior to practicing yoga may be advantageous as it can be a warm-up and once it is done you can turn your focus to yoga. If you are too busy to practice any of this, something needs to change!

**1. Get out of bed before sunrise**

There is uplifting energy freely emanating that can be employed to promote vitality, clarity and synchronization with the waking hours. To remain in bed increases drowsiness.

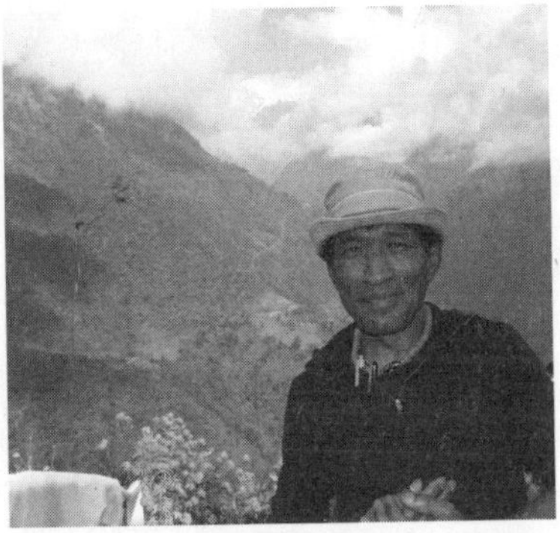

**2. Morning Ablutions**

These practices open and cleanse the 9 Gates of the Body. They include urination, defecation, oral hygiene, visual hygiene, nasal hygiene and auditory hygiene.

Firstly use the toilet and wash your hands.

Perform your oral hygiene practice. If you have ama in the head or neck or imbalance such as cancer, perform oil gandush for 10 minutes three times a day. Oil gandush is also used with mouth ulcers and bleeding gums at vata times, 2-6 AM or PM.

An option for water gandush is to use ¼-teaspoon triphala powder in water. An option for a dentifrice is to use triphala or haritaki powder.

You can appraise the level of ama in your plasma by the amount of it on your tongue day to day.

To equalize the temperature of the mouth with the eyes, while you are rinsing the mouth with water for the last time, touch the same temperature water on your eyelids. While doing so you could consider mentally "On this day may I perceive the Divine in everything I see." You may have already placed flowers, plants, the symbol of your deity or a picture of loved ones to receive as visual nourishment. Or it may be the aliveness in your own eyes you see in the mirror. The first visual impressions of the day are important.

Massage your tongue on all sides. This muscle should feel soft and even. Grasp the tongue with a dry cloth and elongate it out the mouth in all directions. I like it without the cloth, slippery as it is. Also massage your palate as far back as the uvula if comfortable. Elongate your tongue out your mouth and then turn it backwards to touch the uvula and behind. As the tongue is a central muscle, massaging it helps to soften the organs, relieve stiffness in the joints and clarify your energy. And maybe give you a laugh to start the day.

## Oil Your Nostrils.

If your nostrils feel blocked or your lungs feel stagnant or your head feels heavy there is a yoga breathing practice in which a long, slow inhalation is taken through the nose and a short, compressed sneeze-like exhalation is released, also through the nose. This requires intent to draw the abdomen and pelvic floor in quickly on the exhale, emptying about two-thirds of the lungs. Be sure that this is safe for your body. This practice can stimulate the navel area and increase heat. Be sure that this is desired. If any dizziness occurs rest longer between the "sneezes" or discontinue. Sit upright where convenient and begin with six, increasing to 12 and decreasing the length of the inhalation when you are practiced.

To open your auditory gates to the environment place a very small amount of cold-pressed oil on your fingers and massage your ears, making request that "On this day may I sense the Divine speaking through the sounds I hear". My son starts throat singing and laughing even before he gets out of bed.

Perhaps a cup of hot water now or later would be welcome.

Morning ablutions, especially urination and defecation would summon us before anything else and oral ablutions are performed before eating or drinking.

### 3. Abhyanga

There are myriad benefits in applying oil and massaging the skin.

Abhyanga aids the movement of lymph, which supports immunity, decongestion and fluid balance. It aids the circulation, which transports nutrients and wastes. It promotes muscle tone by contact with the muscles through the skin. It releases endorphins, which are natural painkillers and releases tryptophan and serotonin (derived from tryptophan), which are anti-spasmodic and anti-depressant. Massage benefits the endocrine axis, one hormone of which is being investigated as slowing the rate of aging - the longevity idea again. Abhyanga softens and mobilizes ama, helping to move it from the deeper tissues to the organs of elimination and opens the channels for this to happen.

The surface of the skin, tactile in its nature, is an extensive sense organ. Vata dosha is pacified with massage movements that follow its own directions of energy. General guidelines for this are as follows: starting from the head down, apply oil to your crown and then to the entire scalp. Massage and move the scalp with small circles. Massage, press and release the bones of the skull along the entire hairline. 'Wash' your face with oiled hands and press and release gently along the bones of the eyes, cheeks and jaw. Massage your ears that have connections to the whole body. Perform long strokes from neck to navel and then from navel to neck on the front, sides and back of the body. Employ circular movements over joints and around the navel. We become more flexible as our hands endeavor to reach our entire surface area. Massage your arms using the long strokes on long bones and circular movements on joints. Massage and manipulate the bones and muscles of your hands and fingers. Give your hands a reflexology treatment. Employ shorter, back and forth movements with both hands over the abdomen, groin, hips and buttocks. Use long strokes from the navel down and up the thighs. Circle the roundness of the kneecaps and behind the knees. Perform long strokes on the lower legs and round movements on the ankles. Massage and manipulate each foot and toe joint and give the soles of the feet a firm, slow, deep reflexology treatment.

Consult books on marma therapy to include with abhyanga and remember that some of these pressure points were used to inflict deadly harm. When marma points are massaged, pressed and released, it can help rebalance energy pathways, organs and dosha-s. Perhaps advice could be sought from a skilled marma practitioner.

Massaging both sides of the body evenly harmonizes both hemispheres of the brain and unifies energy. To do this, perform as many strokes on the right arm and leg as on the left and where possible use both hands simultaneously on the two sides of the body. As part of ama mobilization, follow the abhyanga with the application of warmth and stay warm for at least 20 minutes.

If the room you are in is cold, only a small portion of the body is uncovered at a time and then recovered after the oil has been massaged in. If the climate is hot, choose a relatively cooler part of the day for massage. Use less friction to avoid increasing heat.

The skin is an organ of consumption. Digestion is aided by pitta dosha present in the skin, which also affects the skin's color and temperature. If a natural product is applied, the body receives the nutrients; if not, the liver has to detoxify it. Massage inhibits hepatic manufacture of cholesterol, lowers blood pressure and helps with emotional release.

Skin is the interface between the individual and the environment. Temperature and dryness can be shielded with oil. Kapha-dominant individuals have natural oil and may feel heavy from too much oil on the skin but still benefit from using a small amount of warmed oil for massage so that the skin is not damaged by dry friction. Afterwards the oil can be removed with mung dal flour or chickpea flour or mild soap during a warm shower or bath. Pitta-dominant individuals have adequate natural oil and use the Part One abhyanga oils for their cooling, grounding effect. They would use massage time for reducing the wound-up nature of pitta-out-of-balance. This helps in staying well. Avoid hot water showers and especially hot water on the head. Vata-dominant individuals luxuriate in the richness of warmed, cold-pressed, cured black sesame oil, as it is more unctuous than white sesame seed oil as well as being heating, nutritious and heavy. Depending on your level of dryness there may be no oil left to shower off. Shower anyway. You may also need to reapply minimal oil after your shower or bath to areas that feel dry.

Leaving excess oil on for more than one hour after self-massage may alter body temperature adversely. It may also increase heaviness and congestion. For the scalp and hair it is recommended to leave a small amount of massage oil distributed so it is best not to use strong detergent shampoos. Traditionally shampoos are not used at all.

The morning toilette may also include combing your hair with a natural comb or brush, shaving and trimming hair and nails.

Following your bath or shower wear clean, natural fiber clothing.

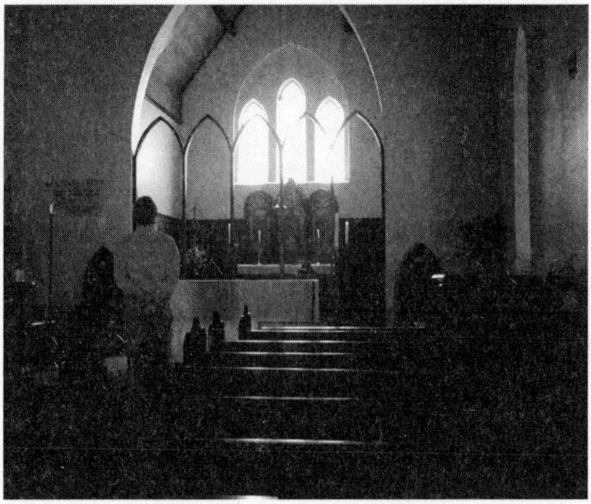

### 4. Meditation - Daily Prayer

Now that you have opened the 9 Gates and showered, you may wish to open the mind channel. One way to prepare is to practice alternate nostril breathing. While seated, tuck the chin in a little towards the throat and lengthen the back of the neck backwards without rounding the back. Fold the index and middle fingers of the right hand halfway towards the palm. Raise the right hand to the nose, keeping the head centered and your right shoulder, elbow and wrist relaxed. Exhale through both nostrils. Close the right nostril with the thumb and slowly, quietly inhale through the left nostril, regulating the amount of air coming in and the time it takes to enter by adjusting the left nostril passage size with the ring finger. It takes very little pressure to manipulate the air passages. Rather than squashing your nostril closed, move your finger to find the cartilage in the vicinity of the nostril crease. Some experimenting will find you the place that takes the least pressure to close the flow of air. Now close the left nostril with the ring finger and release the right nostril to the extent that you can slowly, quietly exhale through it. This is half a round. Inhale through the right nostril and exhale through the left in the manner already described. Continue for up to 12 rounds only if the breathing remains smooth and comfortable. At first sign of distress, stop the pranayama practice and go back to normal, spontaneous breathing. If you persist you will agitate your body and mind.

Meditation in its traditional definition cannot be done, it happens when the mind becomes absorbed through the workings of prana, the forward moving life force. We practice *training* for meditation that cleanses the much-used mental channel. It is ideal to be sitting for training before or at sunrise. One may observe the actual sunrise and flow with that experience for some time. Communion with the highest power is of merit as well.

Over time daily practice will train the moving mind to have more and more periods of uncluttered awareness, non-judgmental discrimination and contentment with what is. The mind will become less habituated to thinking and more habituated to remaining in the present experience. The calmer the mind, the less stress for the body. The tension we feel is mostly the result of mental panic, judgment and worry which creates a friction between what we think should be, what we imagine to be and what truly is. We align with Buddhist teachings when we allow things to be as they are without wanting to squirm out of them or into them. Eventually we come to be in a meditative state without formal practice anymore.

To harness this powerful energy requires some perseverance at first and then becomes a voluntary and satisfying activity. The mind is so ethereal yet exerts such force. Let us remember to make it our wonderful servant, not allow it to be our terrible master.

At this stage you may be enjoying 20 to 60 minutes of practice.

If one feels too heavy or scattered in the mind to practice meditation training first, then practice yoga, tai chi, chi kung or take a walk.

### 5. Yoga/ Tai Chi/ Chi Kung and Exercise

To develop and circulate energy to the whole body, knead the internal organs, align the breath, promote mind-body unity and experience yourself as a multidimensional being, choose from yoga, tai chi, chi kung or similar practices. Between 15 and 30 minutes is beneficial. If the environment is cold or your body feels stiff in the morning, engage in some large body movements to warm up first. Moving the body attentively has, for some people, the same benefits of stress reduction as meditation practice. We use the mind that way too and it's all interconnected anyway.

Kapha-dominant individuals would have a more vigorous physical practice. To overcome their lethargy is the first step. Pitta-dominant individuals would practice yoga or other exercise with the intent to benefit the body rather than use the body for outward appearance and competition. Vata-dominant individuals would sustain physical movements fluidly and hold yoga poses with their muscles active and without overtaxing their energy. In energy-gathering movements, for all people, if the breath is comfortable of its own accord, the practice will be beneficial. If the breath is agitated, short, forced or uncomfortable there is restriction in the system that needs to be investigated. Some of this comes from your sleep from last night, the food you ate and the ama in your system, both physical and mental.

Aerobic exercise is undertaken to provide activation of the heart, circulation, metabolism and body. A 20-minute walk is its simplest and most natural form, adjusting the speed to raise the heart beat to an appropriate rate for you.

### 6. Breakfast

The feeling of hunger is a necessary pre-requisite to eating. If you consistently have low appetite, see the section entitled CULINARY MEDICINE below. Eat breakfast in a pleasant, relaxed setting without mentally jumping ahead into the day. Allow half the space in the stomach for solid food, one quarter for liquids and one quarter to remain unfilled. Include the six tastes in every meal.

### 7. Work, Study and Occupation

Now begins the outward part of the day. Having taken care of yourself on all levels you can interact with others without depleting yourself in the process. The daily routine so far provides and sustains the importance of self-care and brings forth a healthy person who is radiant and loving.

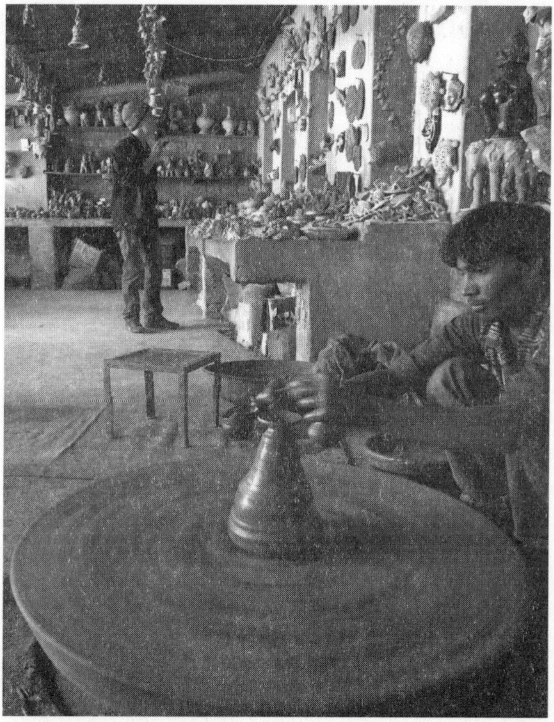

An occupation is most beneficial if it brings satisfaction. We can all recall an experience of helping an adult, child, animal, insect, plant or anything else that left us with a happy, positive feeling. We are all gifted with abilities that are, if possible, used and expressed for the greater good. However, there is no menial assignment in life because every action and interaction is connected with the Divine. Every task is an opportunity for service. When we complain about what we are asked to do, it is a mental judgment by the ego and a reflection of rajas and tamas acting in our mental sphere.

The sattwic mind wants to provide service. The rajasic mind jumps into action and wants what is in its own interest. The tamasic mind is not receptive to any positive growth. Many teachings encourage us to be aware of sattwa as it is the basic nature of mind and acting from there is best for our own health and the benefit of everyone else.

### 8. Midday Meal

Attuned with the strength of the sun in the midday period, our digestive fire is also at its zenith. This is the better time for a complex meal, the largest and heaviest. In summer or in hot weather a light meal may be more appropriate and cooked food is better than raw as the digestive fire is lower in hot weather and raw food needs a strong digestive fire.

After the meal, taken in a relaxed manner and after a short walk, it is good to rest so that the majority of energy can attend to digestion. It is not good to sleep after eating as energy is drawn away and digestion slows down too much leading to formation of ama. If you find that your meal has produced indigestion (see COMPLETE DIGESTION below) perhaps the food chosen was not appropriate for your constitution. Perhaps leftovers were eaten, the meal was too large or your surroundings were unsettled. As natural distress-free digestion is the basis of health, it is worthwhile taking the time to find out how it works best for you and promote it.

### 9. Resume Daily Occupations

While doing what we do during the day, it is important not to suppress natural urges, just as it is important not to be impolite when allowing those natural urges to occur. Ongoing suppression or forcing of the urge to use the toilet, sneeze, yawn, belch, fart, rest, eat, drink or ejaculate produces imbalance.

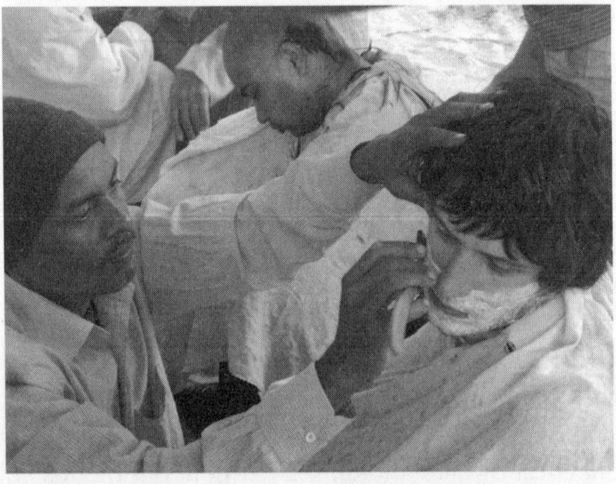

### 10. Late Afternoon

Upon returning home one may perform abhyanga if it was not done in the morning. Late afternoon is a good time to pacify vata dosha with this practice. Eating something grounding such as a healthy unctuous savory or sweet snack would do so as well.

Vata-dominant people can massage often to help prevent vata imbalances, several more of which are dry skin, nervousness and confusion. Pitta-dominant people using coconut oil find relief from windburn, sunburn and heat. A few drops of sandalwood oil can be added to the base oil. Enjoy your self-spa at least two to three times a week. Kapha-dominant people can stimulate their energy and knead their muscles deeply one to three times a week, removing excess oil afterwards as described already.

### 11. Meditation at Sunset

Just as sunrise is a potent time of day, so too is sunset. It is good to attune again with the sun. Being aware of the length of day between sunrise and sunset connects us with the rhythm of the sun over the year. Sitting for meditation or practicing mind-body movements helps release the unevenness of the day's activities and relieves physical stress and mental agitation. If your work is sedentary a more vigorous physical practice may be needed. If you have an active job a more calming practice is better.

The closer it gets to bedtime, the less strenuous the exercise program.

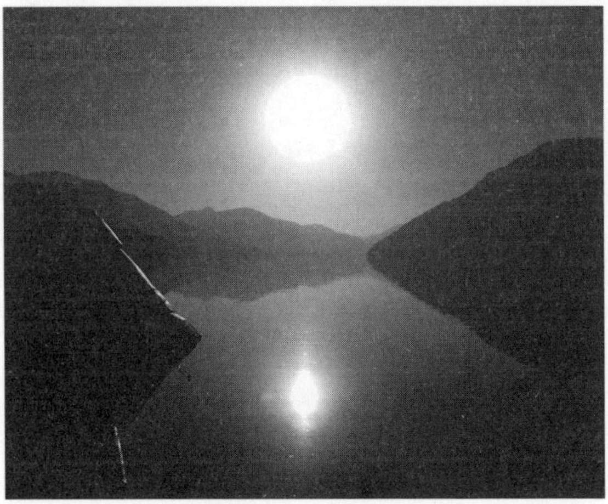

### 12. Light Early Evening Meal

Having enjoyed the majority of the food one eats at the midday meal, and as the sun's fire is no longer apparent if you live in the tropics or temperate zone, evening is the time for a lighter, simpler meal. Even with a vegetarian diet there are several foods that are restricted after sundown, sesame and yogurt being two of them because they are 'heavier', meaning harder to digest.

It is important to have all food out of your stomach by the time you go to sleep. Eating a late dinner encourages ama formation due to incomplete digestion and makes the mind restless or dull the next day. One form that ama takes is excess weight.

A small amount of boiled milk taken with turmeric and nutmeg is acceptable just before bed. If you use saffron, the rich woman's turmeric, it releases its attributes better into water than into full fat milk. Soak a few threads in one tablespoon of warm water for 20-30 minutes before adding to hot milk.

### 13. Short Walk

Having finished any meal, having rested at the table for 5 minutes, having rinsed the mouth, it is helpful to one's digestion to have a short walk. This can be extended if you wish. All digestive walks are for gentle stimulation of the pace of digestion rather than weight loss, fitness, etc.

### 14. Light, Pleasant Activities

During the day we have done work and provided for others in large sweeps of accomplishment. Take time to appreciate the interactions that took place. It is said that to work constantly gives us no time to appreciate our achievements or to assess outcomes and change strategies. Allow the mind to express its thoughts so that it can be assured that what has to be done will be done. Then turn to the free time of the evening.

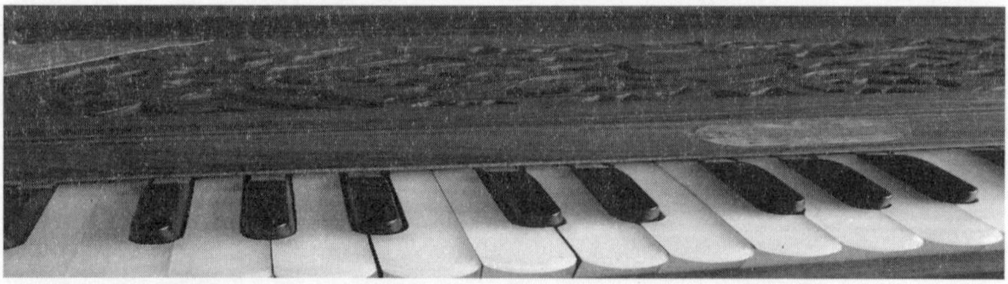

As we near bedtime we wind down our activity. Easy-going conversation with friends and family, meeting with a spiritual group, artistic endeavors, hobbies, reading that will create a favorable impression for dreams, listening to music and homework may be pursued, remembering that we do not wish to over-stimulate the body, mind and senses on most nights.

15. Sex circa 9 PM

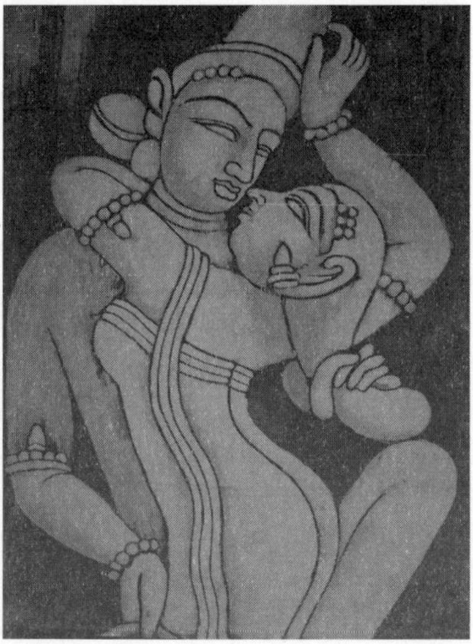

On those nights we do wish to stimulate the body, mind and senses.

16. Sleep circa 10 PM

Sleeping at night is the way we keep our harmony with the rhythm of the sun. Humans are not nocturnal animals. This rhythm varies according to season and latitude. During the night our physical body undergoes cleansing and growth and deep sleep is our primary antioxidant.

At 10 PM we are in transition from a kapha period of time that supports slowing down, stability, softness and heaviness to a pitta period, which will stimulate us again. The longer we remain awake past 10 the more difficult it may be to fall asleep and sleep restfully. If there is not a lot of ama present in the body, going to sleep at this time supports rejuvenation during sleep and an alert, vital start to the next day. If there is a lot of ama, it will interfere with our alignment and use of natural energies. We would hardly expect to feel super great the next morning if we are already carrying the weight of high ama.

The larger one's body mass and the more physically active one's day, the more sleep one will need. The older we are, the less we may require. Between five and eight hours is appropriate. May your rest be healing and restorative and may you awaken refreshed and feeling fine.

Please do your best to maintain a consistent time schedule for having your meals, going to bed and waking up. As our bodies follow a mental clock this will be better for health and rejuvenation. A variation of 30 to 60 minutes day-to-day is acceptable.

## COMPLETE DIGESTION

There are three components to complete digestion, which provide the basis of good health.

### DEEPAN - APPETITE

When we receive the physical sensation of hunger, it is the signal to eat. The body is ready to digest food and food is needed at that time. To eat when we are not hungry can mean there is still food being digested from a previous meal or that the body is digesting ama already present in the gastro-intestinal tract. To burden the system with more food at this time will increase ama. To postpone eating when hungry unsettles the nervous system and weakens the digestive fire, thus disturbing the rest of the body-mind and can lead to future digestive problems. Ayurvedic teachings advise us to eat when we are hungry and not eat when we do not experience actual appetite. Normal digestion will naturally align to mealtimes discussed above in the ayurvedic day.

### PACHAN - DIGESTION

If our food is digesting properly we experience satisfaction. There is no sense of tiredness, nausea, feeling too full, headache, hiccups or stomach gurgling. There is no experience of acidity or heartburn, excess thirst, ravenous appetite, a metallic taste in the mouth or feeling hot. Nor do we feel bloated, experience flatulence or have poor appetite. The tongue is not coated and the nails are smooth without ridges. There are no symptoms that may be called 'indigestion' following a meal.

We can think of our digestive fire (jatharagni) like a campfire we wish to cook over. We start to build the fire slowly with kindling, perhaps a digestive aperitif such as aloe or refer to CULINARY MEDICINE below for suggestion. We avoid smothering the flame with too much fuel, which may occur if we eat too fast, eat too much, eat heavy, oily or leftover food or combine foods in ways that the body cannot digest. We protect the flame from being blown horizontally away from the cooking vessel by using a wind guard, by eating in a relaxed manner, by avoiding iced or cold food or beverage and by avoiding prolonged fasting. We prevent the fire from raging out of control by limiting the accelerant, excessively sour, salty or pungent foods and perhaps using cooling spices and herbs if necessary. As a flame needs oxygen to reach the wood, we allow space in the stomach for the proper mechanical breakdown of food. If a vessel is filled to the brim, it is not possible to mix the contents.

## ANULOMAN - ELIMINATION

If we consume solid food on a daily basis it is necessary to eliminate solid waste once or twice daily. Morning regularity is an important component of health. Solid waste indicates good digestion if it floats, is formed and has the consistency of a ripe banana, is not extremely malodorous, is not sticky, does not contain undigested food, blood or mucus. There is a feeling of complete evacuation without strain and there is no explosive action. In traditional philosophy, the action of elimination is one of life's experiences. We can adjust our diet, working backwards, until we have the perfect evacuation. Sitting on a western toilet, especially for long periods of time, is not conducive to bowel health. Both constipation and diarrhea indicate indigestion and need to be investigated. The pitta constitution does tend towards more unformed stool and several bowel movements each day. Use water instead of toilet paper and dry by absorbing the water with a soft natural fiber cloth.

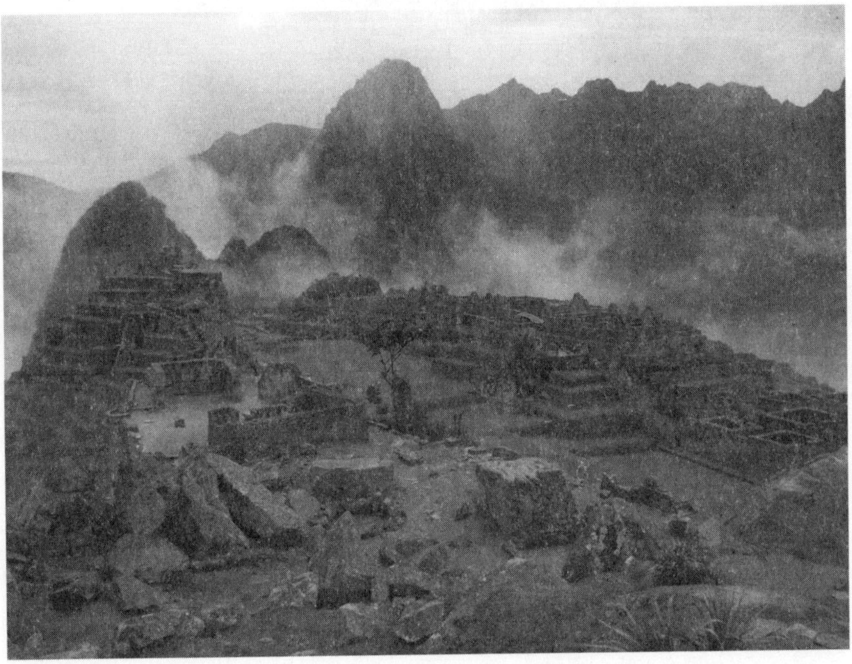

# CULINARY MEDICINE

Ginger (*Zingiber officinale*) and Turmeric (*Curcuma longa*) are from the same family. The aromatic underground stems are used in cooking and to remedy many imbalances.

GINGER is known as the universal remedy. It is an expectorant, increases perspiration, improves digestion and liver function, controls nausea, vomiting and coughing, stimulates the circulation, relaxes spasms, relieves pain and is emmenagogue. It is not used when there is inflammation of skin, digestive tract or fever. Ginger is sweet and pungent, the dried powder more pungent and internally heating, the fresh rhizome promoting perspiration, taking heat outward to the skin.

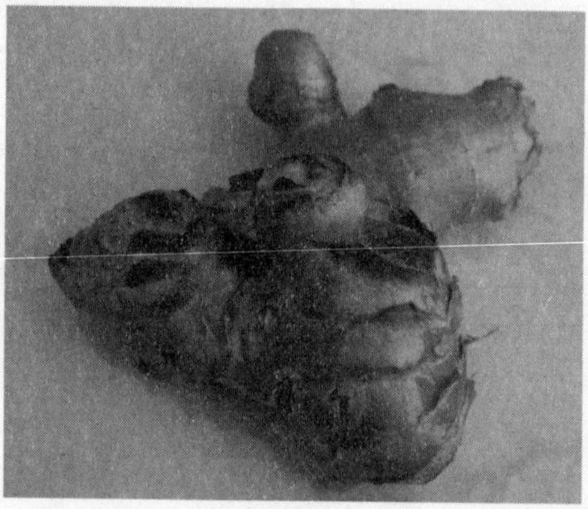

## A FEW APPLICATIONS, APPRAISE HOW THEY WORK FOR YOU

1. Use 1/8-teaspoon powder in hot water as a digestive drink after meals.

2. Dry roast ¼-teaspoon cumin seeds. Add to boiling water with ¼-teaspoon ginger powder. Let cool to drinking temperature and use before meals to decrease bloating.

3. Combine ginger powder, ghee and jaggery in equal amounts. Take ½-1 teaspoon in warm water before meals to improve digestion.

4. Grate 1-teaspoon fresh ginger and infuse in 1-cup boiling water. Cool to body temperature and add 1-teaspoon lemon juice and 1-teaspoon unfired honey. Sprinkle on some fresh ground black pepper. Drink and retire to bed under blankets to allow sweating to dissipate the first signs of cold or flu. Or

drink the tea while you sit wrapped in blankets with your feet in a fresh ginger tea warm bath. Perspire for a short time, them sponge off and use dry clothes and bedding.

5. Spread a thin coat of honey on a piece of cloth and sprinkle with ginger powder. Tape over a painful or congested area. Or make a fresh ginger tea and immerse a piece of fabric in it while still hot. Wring out and place on body where circulation and warmth are required. Cover with plastic and place a heating pad on top.

6. Combine 1-teaspoon ginger powder, 1-teaspoon crushed black peppercorns and 2-teaspoons powdered aniseed. Mix with unfired honey to make a paste. Take ½- teaspoon once or twice a day to alleviate allergies, reduce mucus or with meals as a digestive stimulant. This is a powerfully heating mixture.

TURMERIC provides protection and decongestion for the liver, strengthens the spleen, stimulates the uterus and regulates menstruation, eases PMT and pain, aids digestion, circulation and respiration, normalizes energy flow and lowers cholesterol. It is a plant steroid. It is antibiotic, anti-inflammatory and anti-coagulant. It aids healing of wounds. Turmeric is bitter, pungent, astringent and warming.

Judge these applications' effects on and in your own body:

1. Sprinkle ¼-teaspoon in some boiled milk to help relieve catarrh.

2. Combine ¼-teaspoon each turmeric and ginger powders and add to ½-cup hot milk. Cool and add 1-teaspoon honey. This helps reduce mucus and relieve loss of voice. Does it work better than number one above?

3. Sprinkle a thin slice of fresh turmeric with rock salt and a few drops of lemon juice and eat before meals to promote digestion.

4. Review Part One, weeks 1 and 2 for use of turmeric to relieve sore throat. This can also offset a cold if taken at first signs.

5. Combine turmeric powder with ghee or castor oil and apply topically to help healing and reduce inflammation. Turmeric also helps skin conditions and warts when taken internally in any of the above oral applications.

Using food as medicine means it rebalances our systems. It can also be used as a protective to remain healthy.

## OTHER CULINARY MEDICINES

ASAFOETIDA (*Ferula asafetida*) provides warming therapy, prevents and eliminates gas, bloating and food stagnation. It benefits the liver, spleen and stomach. It calms hysteria. It is pungent and bitter. It initiates a downward movement and can help shift constipation. Decrease over-use during pregnancy. Every serve of beans and pulses is better digested with a sprinkle of 'hing'.

BLACK PEPPER (*Piper nigrum*) is pungent. It is used in warming therapy to stimulate circulation, digestion and metabolism. It helps alleviate constipation, dry hemorrhoids, gas and loss of appetite. It helps dry out mucus. It can be taken with boiled water to induce sweating. It can be mixed with unfired honey and taken in the morning to re-circulate nutrients and also combat worms in the colon. Mixed with ghee it relieves pitta disorders such as hives and dermatitis. It is most beneficial for kapha. Be conservative with this potent spice.

CARDAMOM (*Eletarria cardamomum*) is sweet, pungent, astringent and slightly heating. It aids digestion and expectoration with its warming and anti-mucus properties. Its camphorous, aromatic fragrance clears the mind. Sprinkle the crushed seeds onto fruit to decrease mucus. As a digestive or expectorant tea combine 4 cups water with 1 bay leaf. Bring to boil and simmer 10 minutes. Remove from heat and add 1 teaspoon each of ginger powder, cinnamon or cassia bark powder and cardamom powder. Cover and infuse for 5 minutes. Sweeten if desired. Try it instead of coffee at a dinner party. Seeds can be chewed after meals to alleviate indigestion. For night time indigestion steep seeds in hot water and drink.

CLARIFIED BUTTER (*ghee*) is sweet, cool and unctuous. It promotes memory, intelligence, digestive fire, semen, immunity and body tissues. It treats inflammation of the gastro-intestinal tract, ulcers and fevers and acidity. It is tonic, soothes the nerves and lubricates tissues and joints. It improves voice and complexion. It is not inherently prone to raise normal cholesterol levels and does not increase pitta heat even though it is an accelerant to digestion.

DATES (*Phoenix dactylefera*) are sattwic, sweet, heavy and cooling. They build the body and support vata and pitta. Add a bit of ghee or oil to the surface of the date to help digest its heavy nature.

FENUGREEK (*Trigonella foenum-graecum*) is contraindicated during pregnancy and approved for lactation. It decreases joint pain. It is both warming and cooling, being pungent and bitter. This combination helps digestion and healing of the GI tract.

JAGGERY (*Saccharum officinale*) is unrefined, solidified cane sugar. It can also be the name for unrefined, solidified palm sap (*Palmyra borassus-flabelliformis*). It is sweet, mildly laxative, calming pitta and vata. It increases marrow, fat and flesh and overuse can increase intestinal worms.

LEMON and LIME (*Citrus sp.*) are sour. The sour taste improves appetite and digestion. These fruits can help reduce liver congestion and acidity but need to be used with caution in pitta conditions. If you experience bloating, reduce the sour taste as it may hold excess fluid in the stomach.

NEEM (*Azadirachta indica*) is bitter and astringent. It is anti-bacterial and anti-inflammatory. It helps control sugar and fat metabolism for kapha and heat for pitta. Being so cooling, it is only good for vata in small doses when needed. It can be applied locally to boils or red and hot skin conditions.

SALT helps to liquefy phlegm and relieve congestion. A mild solution of salt water cleanses the mouth, throat and nose to relieve mucus. It softens food for digestion and relieves gas and distention of the abdomen. To relieve external swelling heat some salt in a pan and place in a cloth bag to apply over the area. Most salts are heating but rock salt used in small amounts is cooling and does not promote water retention. Therefore it is appropriate for all constitutional types in normal quantity.

TULSI, the sacred basil plant (*Ocimum sanctum*), is warming and has a refreshing fragrance and sattwic properties. A tea made with the leaves relieves cough, colds, headache and fever and improves stamina. If the leaves are mixed with ginger it relieves stomach disorders.

# FOOD WISDOM

## AVOID SOME FOODS AND FOOD COMBINATIONS:

Dairy and salted food

Dairy and animal food, especially fish

Milk is best on its own but can be taken with grains

Fruit and other food

Very cold and very hot food taken together

Mixing fresh and leftover food

The proportion of 3 parts ghee and 1 part honey

Never heat honey, buy only unfired, unprocessed honey

Milk and honey

Yogurt, cheese, sesame and other heavier foods at night

A steady diet of alkaline food

Microwaved, preservative-laced and GE foods

Processed foods, refined foods, artificial flavors, colors

Freezing (prana cannot be frozen and freezing makes things harder to digest)

Raw foods as a steady diet: 25% of food intake per day is fine

Fermented foods (interferes with kapha and pitta zones of digestion—Cultured foods are fine)

Fried foods (heavy, acid residue in stomach)

Excess sugar and salt

Carbonation (hyperactivity of GI tract, and these drinks usually cold)

Overly spiced food (excess heat and restless mind)

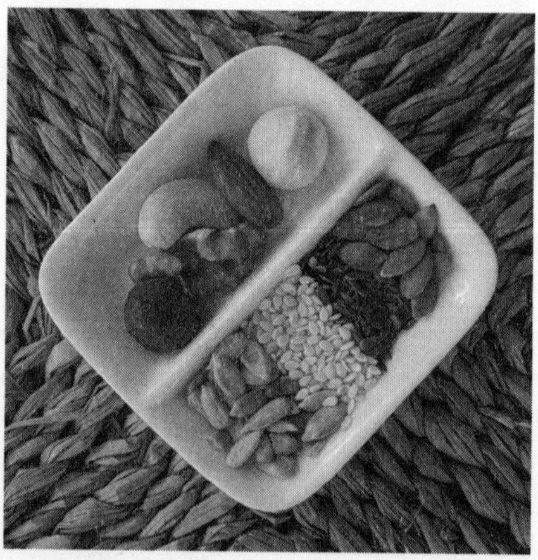

## SOME FOOD BALANCERS:

**Cheese**: black pepper or trikatu mix (black pepper, long pepper, ginger)

**Eggs**: parsley, coriander, turmeric, cooked onions

**Ice cream or sour cream**: cloves, cardamom or coriander powder

**Yogurt**: cumin or ginger powder and at lunchtime only

**Legumes**: black pepper, ginger, turmeric, asafoetida, rock salt, lemon

**Cruciferous vegetables**: turmeric, mustard seed, can also use cumin and ajowan seed

**Banana**: cardamom

**Raw salad**: olive oil and lemon juice dressing

**Potato**: ghee with black pepper

**Tomato**: cumin

**Avocado**: turmeric, lemon, garlic if using, black pepper

**Dry fruit**: soak

**Melon**: coriander

**Alcohol or chocolate**: chew cumin or cardamom seeds

**Black tea**: add milk and ginger or chai spice mix, can add sugar if desired

**Caffeine and coffee**: nutmeg with cardamom

**Popcorn**: add ghee

**Sweets**: ginger powder

**Tobacco**: celery seeds

**Bread**: toast it

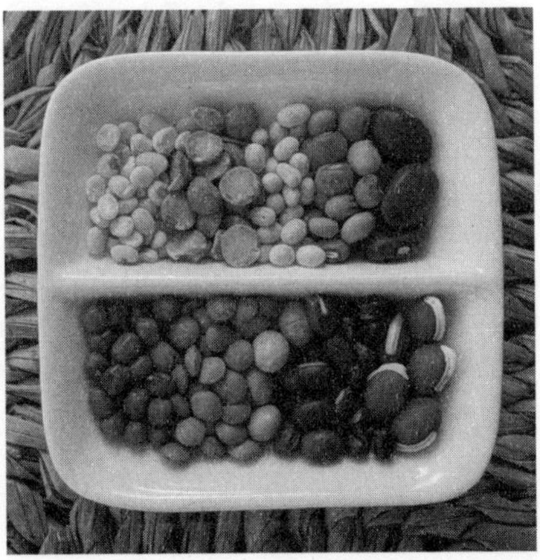

# MOTHER and CHILD HEALTH

Let us begin with female puberty and make a full circle to the health of all adolescents.

## PUBERTY AND MENSTRUATION

The proper menstrual cycle is 28-30 days with a 4-day bleed to remove all impurities from the uterus. If a woman bleeds less there is incomplete cleansing and the impurities will remain until the next period, making it more taxing. The flow should be neither heavy nor light.

## SOME ADOLESCENTS BLEED HEAVILY BECAUSE

1. their diet is not good and includes the consumption of too much meat
2. they take heavy exercise
3. they are overweight
4. they are stressed and their mental health is poor

## SOME BLEED SCANTILY BECAUSE

1. their food is irregular or drying and light. Some will have skin problems in this category because the impurities of the blood, naturally removed with a normal bleed, are not removed.
2. they take heavy exercise. A woman should not participate in sports during her period.
3. they are underweight
4. they are stressed and their mental health is poor

We all need good food. Food habits to cultivate are the same for everyone: freshly cooked, warm, slightly unctuous food, with the six tastes to create vata, pitta and kapha in equilibrium and of good quality. Stop eating after a good burp (odorless), or when you feel full and refreshed. With too much food, there will be many burps, a feeling of heaviness, sweating, eyes watering and feeling sleepy. Eating less is also not good as it weakens jatharagni (not enough food to sustain the function of the digestive fire).

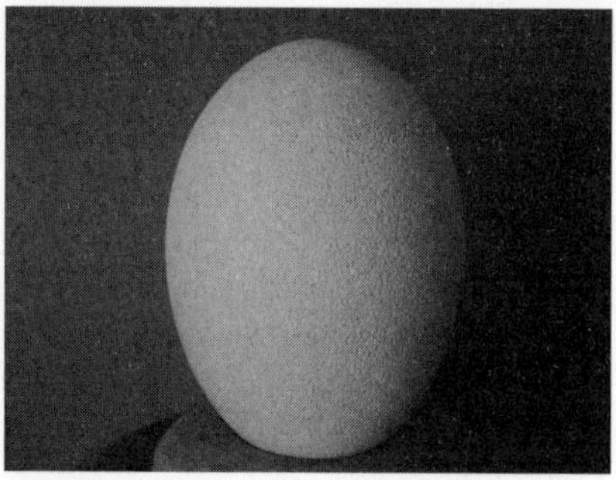

Two common ayurvedic herbs, both tonic to the uterus, are shatavari and ashwagandha powders. These are sweet and supportive herbs. They are roots that need a good digestion to process them. The taste of the remedy is a signal to the body so with all remedies please allow the taste to be tasted. In my early ayurveda days I used to imbed the remedy, try to hide it in food. The kids tasted it anyway and I felt my actions had been underhanded.

There is a correlation between pain and a scanty bleed. If there is pain and cramps, abhyanga over the abdomen and lower back with a warm pack afterwards may help. Do not do a total body massage during your menstrual period because it retards the flow. The teachings would also recommend an oil basti, which is a quarter cup warm sesame oil (cold-pressed, organic, cured) given as a rectal enema. Do not introduce air with the oil. Rest for 15 minutes. What is not absorbed will be excreted when nature calls. This is calming vata to the seat of vata. If you do this about 4-5 PM you will increase the effects even more.

| DOSHA AFFECTED | PRE-MENSTRUAL | MENSTRUAL |
|---|---|---|
| Vata | Nervous tension<br>Mood swings<br>Anxiety<br>Depression<br>Insomnia<br>Forgetfulness<br>Constipation<br>Bloating<br>Fatigue<br>Tension headaches | Pain<br>Cramps<br>Back ache<br>Cramping in legs<br>Extended bleed<br>Light flow<br>Dark, clotted blood<br>Irregular spotting |
| With menopause | Acceleration of anxiety, fear, worry, insecurity, dryness of skin, membranes and bones | |

| DOSHA AFFECTED | PRE-MENSTRUAL | MENSTRUAL |
| --- | --- | --- |
| Pitta | Irritability and anger<br>Increased appetite<br>Sugar cravings<br>Migraines<br>Excessive sweating<br>Feeling of excess heat<br>Diarrhea or increased bowel movement<br>Rashes and acne | More bleeding<br>Frequent bleeding such as every 2 weeks<br>Sudden onset of migraine especially around the eyes |
| With menopause | More heat, anger, irritation and mood swings | |
| Kapha | Weight gain<br>Fluid retention<br>Breast enlargement or engorgement<br>Lethargy<br>Vaginal Candidiasis<br>Slow digestion | Stiffness in back or joints<br>Pale, mucus-like flow<br>Pale mucoid clots<br>Endogenous depression |
| With menopause | Weight gain, fluid retention and depression | |

## CAREER AND EARLY ADULTHOOD

The best contraception is knowing your own cycle and using a physical barrier such as a condom. Any change in your life can change your cycle.

If your gift is being good at sports, if sport expresses your true nature, pursue it. We spectators thank you for inspiring us with what the mind-body is capable of. Be aware that it will be difficult to keep your menstrual cycle working well. We know that female athletes become amenorrheal. This means that whilst the exercise is promoting a good (or excessive) rate of metabolism, the uterus is not getting cleansed nor is the blood. If our reproductive hormones and organs are not functioning, the feminine gender strength is reduced.

Make conscious choices throughout the month to promote a life in balance. Create routine in tune with the natural cycles of day and night. In the week prior to your period, in addition to an occasional or more frequent bowel cleanse, mix together 1-teaspoon fresh ginger juice and 1-teaspoon unprocessed honey in warm water and consume once a day. This is a very potent detoxifier and also very heating. If you run hot, please pass on this. Once you are feeling lighter and clearer and your menstrual periods are working well, you can discontinue this drink.

All practices, natural and modern, have a bearing on pregnancy, delivery, your sons' and daughters' health and on your health. Oral contraception, IVF and even endometriosis have a bearing on the uterine environment.

## RAISING A FAMILY

Diet, lifestyle and ama in the body will affect the fertility of the couple and strength of the sperm and ovum, which affects the child's prakruti. Both parents would spend 6-12 months lessening their ama and increasing their nutrition and peace of mind before trying to conceive.

With the imbalance of infertility, an ayurvedic doctor would consult at length about each person's overall health including the strength of the digestive fire. Infertility means the essence of the food we eat is not moving through the first six tissues to the seventh, the reproductive tissue. Also know that alcohol is "pure sour" and the sour taste increases all body tissues except the reproductive tissue. That, it decreases.

There are many herbs and preparations that strengthen the uterus, the ova, the sperm and semen and several gentle procedures to cleanse the uterus and oleate the surrounding tissues. Fertility was always high priority in India, what with the maharajas wanting many strong sons.

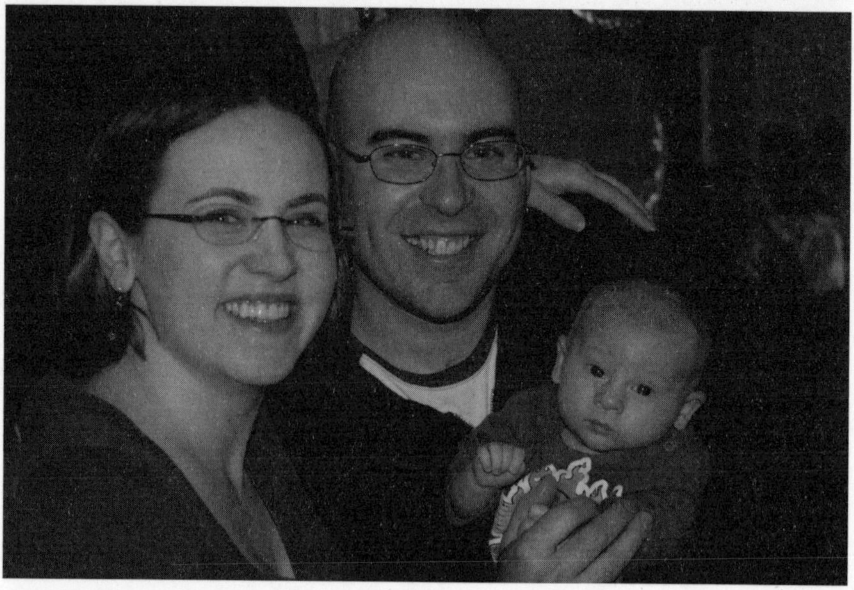

## PREGNANCY

The best years for commencing motherhood are between 25-35 years of age, when a woman's body and mind are neither unstable as one can be in youth nor rigid as one can become later on. It is best to avoid travel as much as possible and extreme exercise when pregnant. Gentle yoga stretches and walking are good. Also avoid being over-sedentary. Enjoy good nutrition with freshly cooked meals using fresh foods and drink an adequate amount of pure water. If you take drugs, recreational or otherwise, consider that they will affect your baby. The mother-to-be needs to be nurtured on all levels and impart that to her developing little one. Contemplate beauty in all forms. Don't watch unsettling films!

The following postures are considered safe for beginner yogini-s during pregnancy and need to be comfortable if you choose to practice them. Please do not bend or extend beyond comfort. Lengthen your torso front and back. Stay in the postures for shorter periods of time. Make sure your breathing is free and steady. Keep your belly relaxed. Although we treat ourselves gently, pregnancy still allows us to be stretched and strong. Our awareness needs to recognize if our joints and ligaments are getting too loose and then not stretch as far. Join a yoga class for pregnant moms, the friendships are long lasting.

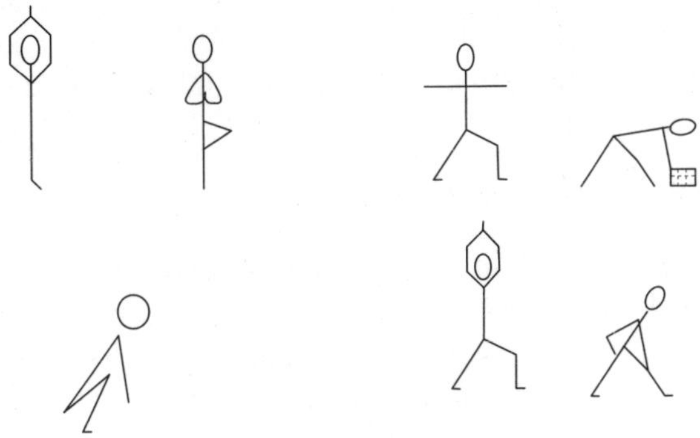

## REST

How do you feel most relaxed while lying…on your side? On your back? With your legs up on the lounge? This will change with your changing body. Bring awareness to each part of you, softening and opening. Do this morning, afternoon, evening or whenever needed. Resting may be the most under-used skill we have.

## BREATHING

In a lying or seated position (on a chair with a uplifting spine is fine or on a recliner if comfortable) become aware of your breathing. Allow the rib cage to lift and widen slowly and evenly on your inhales, allow your ribs and abdomen to relax with your exhales. This is also practice for lactation as oxygen goes into making milk. You are breathing for two but please do not hyperventilate and become light-headed.

## MEDITATION

Pregnancy is a perfect time to bring your mind into focus on your changing body and the life within. You can sing to your baby, share the life force with your baby as you breathe, share a sense of beauty, welcome, awe and joy.

## BIRTH

The birth process is a high-energy event, under the direction of Mother Nature. It is an experience of pure presence. Allow yourself to be the instrument that nature is playing. It is possible to lie on your side, sit on a birthing stool or be on all four's. If you experience the urge to push, then do, and then rest. For my second home birth I let the contractions do the pushing. Feeling safe is important. This is no time to negotiate the particulars. Choose a birthing team who will attend to your every whim and cheer you on.

## POST NATAL

What happens after the birth of your baby can influence you in later stages of life.

New mothers, apply the following as much as possible.

1. Rest after delivery. The energy of movement, in this case the downward movement of birth, has drawn from the reservoir of overall energy and needs to be replenished. Sleep whenever possible as you will be up at all hours of the day and night until motherbaby forms a routine. One friend said to her second child, "Dear one, you must have longer sleeps at night." And the baby did!

2. Take care of vata with warm gentle sesame oil massage. If desired you can use gentle steaming of the body but not the head. Stay out of bad weather. When vata is disturbed, mental health is disturbed.

3. Yoga consists of supine resting and breathing only. It is still yoga when you are present in it.

4. Get all the blood out of the uterus to prevent toxaemia or curettage; use heating herbs such as ginger and black pepper in your food.

5. Lactation needs good nutrition as did pregnancy, so include in your diet red, black or ordinary dates, peeled soaked almonds and white poppy seeds. Also use cumin seeds and ghee.

6. Bring best quality milk to boil, cool and add some jaggery- unrefined cane sugar- and cardamom. Soak saffron in warm water and add to milk and food.

7. Any breast milk that your baby spits up may be due to the foods you are eating. Babies can be so discerning as to like it when mom eats red apples and not like it when she eats yellow apples. Mothers: eating stewed fruit will be better for baby.

8. A quarter cup of warm (cold-pressed, organic, cured) sesame oil as a rectal enema is good for the uterus. Take three in that first month. Rest 10-15 minutes afterwards, what is required will be absorbed, the rest is eliminated. Do not introduce air with the oil. Dashamoola taila is sesame oil with grounding herbs; use it instead of sesame oil if you have access to it. You can make an espichoo, an organic cotton homemade tampon

impregnated with dashamoola oil instead of an enema. Let it remain 1-2 hours in the vagina, it is faster acting than the enema and helps reduce fibroids.

9. Yoni dhavan is a vaginal douche with herbs to flush the uterus. There is also yoni dhoopan which is squatting over herbal smoke.

10. In India mother and child stay indoors for 45 days at her mother's, where the new mother is protected, safe and has no chores. This helps prevent post-natal depression. The first outing is to the temple where the child is put in front of god. One's parents are the sine qua non of one's life (without which not) and are always cherished.

11. At home the family unit needs re-enforcing, with the father included and supportive. The mother needs three quality fresh warm meals cooked for her each day, eaten in peace, boiled milk if she is tolerant to it and rest to help herself and baby. This is the best thing she can give her child.

12. Baby can sleep next to the parents' bed in a futon hammock, which holds baby like the womb.

## INFANT HEALTH-FIRST TRIMESTER

**First trimester of life requires the most care for mother and child.**
**Routine for baby**: First, massage your baby with sesame/coconut oil blend. Sesame is heating, coconut is cooling so the proportion depends on climate and season. The frontal bones of the head are massaged which helps brain nutrition. Massage a good amount of oil in the ears, nose and anus, which helps ground these openings dominated by vata. Put a cotton ball soaked in oil on the anterior fontanel and cover the baby's head with a cap. Massage helps your baby recuperate from the birth process and can be done everyday for up to three years if the child stays still. Oil for hands, arms, legs and feet is called chandan bala, which develops strong bones. Use it instead of sesame/coconut oil if you have access to it. (This oil helps in arthritis or bone pain, especially as guggul for adults.)

**Second, exercise your baby, moving his or her limbs.**

**Third**, bathe in warm to comfortably hot water. For the first 3 months wash your baby with the following if you wish: finely grate and soak half a peeled almond in pure water while you massage your baby and use it as almond "milk". Certainly use no soap. Dress baby in warm clothes with a tight wrap.

**Fourth**, feed your baby. The above procedures have ignited the digestive fire and baby should be hungry.

**Finally, put your baby to sleep. This whole routine will help the child grow.**

Do this around 8-9 AM and in the evening for the first few months and avoid letting the baby get cold. Even in summer keep your baby warm but not overheated.

**Baby milk formula**: if you are or are not breast-feeding and/or if baby wants more and is not ready for solids (5 months old at least), use the following mix instead of commercial formulas. Mix half pure water, half best quality cow's milk, the smallest amount of organic ginger and turmeric powders and vidanga powder (*Embelia ribes*) if available and bring to a good boil. A small amount of organic sugar can be added. Milk is a saline product and needs no salt. Cool and feed to your baby.

Babies are not given just water to drink before 4 months of age. Prior to four months guti is given, an herbal concoction in mother's milk that balances the baby's dosha-s. The first water that is given is the excess water in which rice has been cooked. The amount is between one teaspoon and one tablespoon at a time. Any food other than mother's milk is considered a foreign substance to baby and must be introduced slowly. This topic is discussed in the next section. The next water can be that which both rice and split mung beans have been cooked in.

If your baby experiences bloating or colic soak a cloth in warm castor oil, apply on belly and cover. This will reduce vata, which is showing up as excess wind. If both parents have cleansed before conceiving, bloating is usually not a problem.

If your infant is constipated, sterilize some soft thin cotton string, wring out, then dip a 1½-inch length into castor oil and insert tenderly in the anus until normal evacuation eliminates it.

**Young babies with skin problems**: check detergent and other sources of allergens. The rash can sometimes be due to emotional factors. What's the tone like at home? Grate some fresh turmeric and mix with mother's milk. Pat this on your child's skin, being aware that turmeric stains permanently. Try to gauge the volume of urine. If your baby is dehydrated it could affect his or her skin.

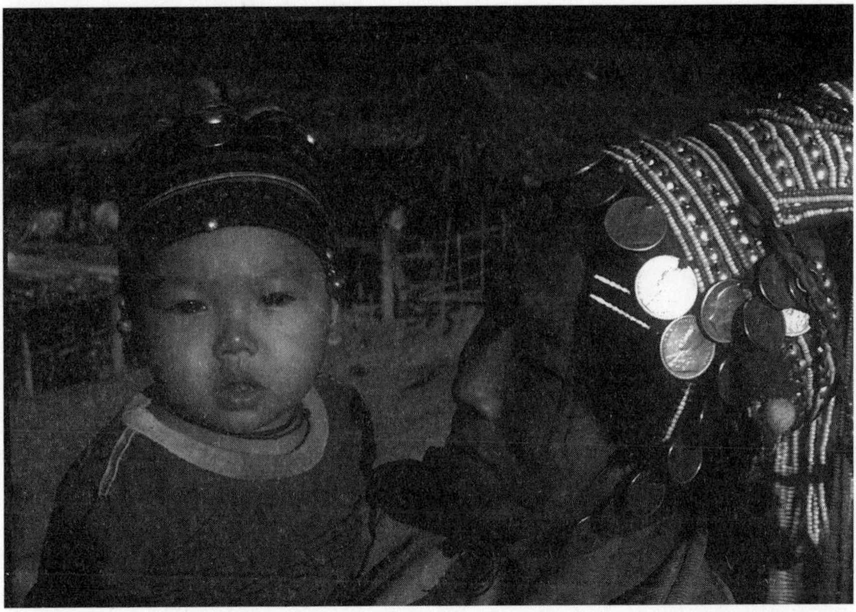

## FIVE MONTHS ONWARD

At this time food can be introduced while still breastfeeding, which can continue up to about one year, longer if desired. If you haven't done so already, first offer the water from cooked rice or split mung beans, between 1 teaspoon and 1 tablespoon.

**Second**, offer the water from cooked vegetables, especially bottle gourd, zucchini, potato, carrot, sometimes pumpkin but not yet beetroot water. Add a wee bit of rock salt, sugar and cumin powder.

**Third**, mash the above well-cooked vegetables with your fingers so that it is more textured than 'baby food' and season as above. This is so that the child develops chewing function. After a week add a small amount of well cooked moist rice and mung to the vegetables, finger-mashed. Serve this twice a day.

Another easily digested food is cooked semolina porridge. To prepare this roast a small amount of semolina in a small amount of ghee (butter oil, not butter), add equal amounts milk and water, bring to boil and cook. Add a small amount of organic sugar and cardamom powder. For these young infants we are talking only a few drops of ghee per meal. This porridge can be breakfast and/or dinner.

**Fruit**: start with seasonal fruit and offer a small amount of its juice. Next, cook the fruit and serve with sweetener. Sometimes fruit is the cause of cough and cold so be aware. Avoid bananas in winter (and rainy season) and when they are eaten in summer add ghee and cardamom. Bananas are a favorite offering by parents but they are hard to digest, hence the ghee and spice.

**Milk**: from an ayurvedic point of view we should develop in children the habit of drinking milk. From one year of age until teenage years 1-cup of milk twice a day is recommended. It should always be heated to boil, cooled, never cold, and have a sprinkle of cardamom and/or turmeric stirred in. Traditional medicines, both Indian and Chinese, remind us that yes, cooking does reduce some enzymes, etc., but provides a food that is easier to digest and assimilate. Indian people as a population have the enzyme lactase to break down milk sugar. Maybe you do not.

**Nuts**: Wait until your child has all his or her baby teeth before introducing nuts. Crack open a few almonds, soak them several hours, peel and serve as almond pieces. This is a good choice. Sunflower and pumpkin seeds freshly hulled are also good.

**Meat and other non-vegetarian food**: do not offer before 2½-3 years of age, it will cause heaviness (tamas) in the physical and mental development of the child. Start with the broth of chicken, then the flesh itself in a soup. Good spices to include are asafoetida (hing), rock salt, turmeric and cumin. These help digest the food.

If an older child is weak or thin, build their digestion as if they are just starting to eat for the first time, that is first rice water, mung water, etc.

If toilet training is slow, sit your child on the toilet in the morning and let them stay for awhile. Very sweet water will stimulate peristalsis. Nappies may mask the connection so keep them out of nappies as much as possible.

Children should have their ears and head covered in cold, rainy or windy weather and wear a cotton undershirt close to their chest until at least 6 years of age. With upper respiratory imbalance massage small children with a coconut and sesame oil blend and put a warm pack on the chest. A woollen undershirt is better for children prone to URI imbalance.

For washing your older infant mix mung bean flour, milk and a bit of freshly grated turmeric. Use fresh turmeric for purity or use organic dried turmeric. Massage into skin and then rinse them in warm water.

**Ringworm and fungal infections**: use triphala (a common ayurvedic herbal preparation) and vidanga in equal amounts with milk or honey; also triphala with ghee and a small amount of sugar.

## PROTECT YOUR CHILD FROM INDUCED ASTHMA

The young child still has an immature digestive system. Sometimes it works, sometimes it is weak. If s/he appears plumper and rosier than usual and if his/her frontal bone protrudes, if there is loss of appetite and an odor on the breath, your child will probably get 'sick' suddenly. There will be a dry cough and the feeling that s/he can't breathe. There will be mucus, which comes out in the stool and/or perhaps by vomiting, and a fever develops to dry it.

If antibiotics are given, the symptoms will be masked and the whole scenario will recycle every 3 weeks. Mask it enough and the child will become asthmatic.

What is happening is that due to the immature digestive system, excess mucus as a waste product is being formed. That is to say the digestion is backing up and it is normal that there is yet not enough fire to digest food efficiently.

To reduce the waste mucus naturally, to bolster immunity and to increase the digestive fire, add turmeric and ginger, one teaspoon each, into ½-cup quality milk (goat or cow) plus ½-cup quality water. Bring to boil. Then cool to body temperature and give your child 1-tablespoon at a time mixed with unfired, unheated honey. Do this 3-4 times in the day. What is not consumed by your child on the day is fine for you to drink that evening if you take milk. In addition, if your child is hungry, decrease all mucus-forming foods and hard-to-digest foods, e.g. all dairy including milk, wheat, nuts and peanut butter (not an ayurvedic recommendation at any time), raw foods including fruit, especially bananas. Boiled rice with mung dal and vegetables and spices outlined above are suitable.

If you are breastfeeding exclusively and this scenario occurs, mother drinks the mucus-reducing drink, eats a mucus-reducing diet and takes care of baby while s/he is processing the imbalance. Of course we are always cautious when fever is a factor.

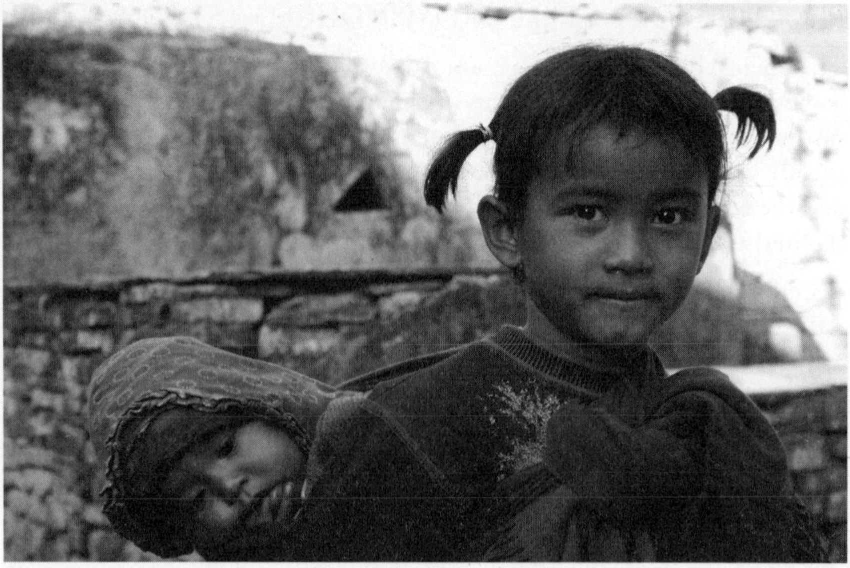

## SCHOOL-AGE CHILDREN

Your child needs energy provided by three cooked meals a day, milk twice a day, vegetables, carbohydrates, protein, good quality oils and less meat. Fruit is a good snack but not as an alternative to a proper cooked meal. Use whole fruit to make unchilled fruit juice slush and add some ginger or cinnamon. This can be diluted with water.

The digestive capacity develops with eating so we want to acclimate our child's digestion to all foods. Start by introducing small amounts, so that digestion will not get too sensitive. We still want to minimize junk food, chocolate and cheese whilst introducing a variety of foods so that allergies do not occur. One cause of allergies is that the child has not been slowly acclimated to the particular food or that his/her digestion was too immature when the food was first offered, usually as an amount that overwhelmed their digestive ability.

Your child can drink warm water. Warming it prevents a startled stomach. Fruit juices are not an alternative to pure water. Some water can also be taken with meals, in total 3-4 cups per day.

Include the 6 tastes in each meal with a predominant sweet taste (which is found in carbohydrate, protein, natural sugars, healthy oils) to promote growth. The sweet taste provides for increase in weight in people of all ages.

**Digestive Upsets**: Children of school age are prone to contracting worms. The herbal powder vidanga helps eliminate them. Use ¼-teaspoon twice a day after meals mixed in warm water until symptoms disappear.

**Diarrhea/dehydration**: Lemonade with a sprinkle of rock salt and ginger powder can be given. No food, as in fever, until appetite returns.

**Ringworm**: Ringworm symptoms include sticky stools and stomach aches especially after meals. If these symptoms are present give your child (who is at least two years of age) a castor oil cleanse once a month until symptoms are gone. Use ¼- ½-teaspoon oil. Children will not necessarily balk at this low dose. Regular castor oil cleansing can commence from 5-6 years of age, once every month or every other month. Start with ½-teaspoon in food or juice. Continue this dose up until about 12 years. This helps with de-worming on a regular basis.

**URI**: Use hot herbs like ginger, black pepper and pippali (long pepper if available) with unfired honey for school age children. This dries out the mucus by increasing the digestive fire. Keep the chest warm. If the child is asthmatic, massage chest with sesame oil and put on a warm-hot pack. Have your child wear a woollen undershirt. Merino wool is very soft on the skin. After massage give a purgative like triphala, which may be vomited out, that's OK as it is getting rid of the mucus. Keeping your child's nasal passages oleated with sesame oil or sometimes ghee may help in preventing infection and allergy.

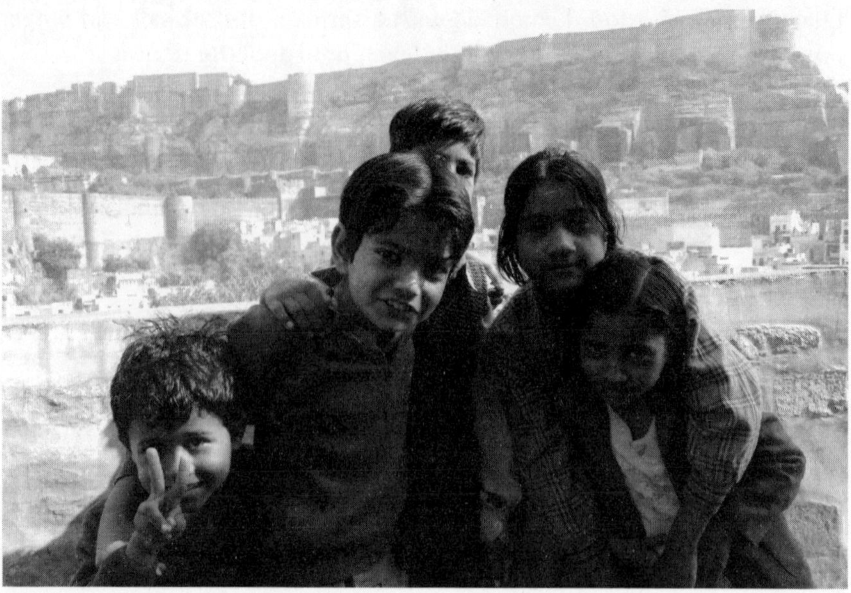

## ADOLESCENCE

The fire component is increasingly active during puberty and adolescents become more strong-headed and short-tempered. We rely on ourselves as parents to practice patience, tolerance and understanding, as children need emotional support at this time of transition.

**Acne**: The powders of manjishta and anantamool are both excellent. Others powders include turmeric and red chandan (sandalwood). Make a thin paste, apply to the skin and let dry. Then wash off. Include turmeric in meals as it is good for everyone. Any of these powders can be warmed in clarified butter and the medicated ghee used if the pimples and skin are dry. The Unani syrup called Safi is a blood and intestinal cleanser. As acne is an indication of ama in both those areas, Safi can help reduce it.

To decrease acne, include enough exercise to counteract stagnation and women, avoid excessive exercise, which can adversely affect the menstrual cycle. Diet would include more vegetables and less meat. Some meat is appropriate if the adolescent is engaged in body-building, sport and other physical workouts, as like increases like, but meat is heating and produces more ama if digestion is not working efficiently.

What children eat outside the home is not under our control, however we can provide nutritious home meals with heaps of love. Many adolescents will minimise junk food if they are made aware of the link between it and how they look and feel. If the habit of eating fruits and vegetables is established early on, your children will continue to do so to some extent throughout life.

Explain to your daughters the advantages and responsibilities of being female and of keeping the uterus healthy. Encourage them to rest during their periods with parents setting the example of mother resting, others cooking and cleaning. Once ama develops in this stage, digestion suffers and long-term imbalance may occur. Encourage a self-massage or professional massage once a week.

**Fever**: Consult a medical practitioner to make sure the fever is not indicative of a serious condition.

The digestive fire has been thrown to the skin so your child will not be hungry. Wait until he or she is hungry to feed and rebuild digestion slowly. Serve soups with rock salt. Asafoetida, turmeric and some ajwan can be added. Do not serve fresh or dried fruit, juices or nuts.

If this is kapha fever with vomiting mucus, cough and cold, a sprinkle of black pepper, ginger and ground aniseed in equal amounts is also helpful. Other symptoms of kapha fever are mucus in the bowel eliminations, sweat on the body and body temperature not too high but remaining elevated a long time.

Cool a pitta fever by wiping room temperature water on the skin. Its temperature is high and symptoms include an acidic or burning feeling, yellow vomit and diarrhea. Make sure you have consulted a health professional for their opinion.

A vata fever fluctuates in temperature as does the child's energy and appetite. Respond according to those fluctuations.

Rest at least one day after the fever is gone. When appetite is good, your child is better.

Avoid exposure to cold and wind.

This completes the recommendations for birth through adolescence.

# INTESTINAL CLEANSE

Clearing the intestines of ama promotes dosha balance. It assists absorption because if the small intestine villi are coated with stagnant material, assimilation cannot take place. This is one reason for malnutrition and eating more in this case will put a larger burden on the body.

The large intestine is responsible for absorption as well. It is said that this is where the vitality (prana) of well-digested food is taken up. If there are toxins accumulating here, that is what is absorbed through the natural function of the bowel and we keep circulating our wastes.

The liver has many functions that help digestion and detoxification. It produces bile salts that reduce fat globules into more assimible size. It stores glucose as glycogen to keep our blood sugar level within healthy range. It is the hottest running organ of the body and does not need more heat in the form of anger, impatience or myriad desires that do not get fulfilled.

The classic cleanse for these organs as well as the pancreas and lower stomach is called virechana, part of panchakarma. The ayurvedic doctor uses natural herbs and methods to flush them. Another over-the-counter purgative is Epsom Salts which is stronger and more dehydrating than ColoZone or castor oil.

A liver cleanse that is used by herbalists in recent times is as follows: for one week prior to the cleanse, drink one glass of fresh apple juice a day to soften any accretions.

On the day of the cleanse enjoy only fat-free food and have your final meal at 4 PM. At 6 PM take 1-teaspoon of ColoZone with lemon juice as outlined in Part One, Weeks 37 & 38 and another teaspoon at 8 PM. Continue to drink warm water during this time.

Just before 10 PM prepare yourself for bed with your evening ablutions. Then mix together ½-cup quality olive oil and ½-cup fresh grapefruit juice. Shake until the oil is emulsified in the juice like a salad dressing (which it is). Stand by your bed and drink it upright within 5 minutes. Lie down with your head high on a pillow and be still for 20 minutes, keeping your stomach area open to facilitate the bile duct opening. You may experience heat or sounds from your internal organs. Go to sleep. If you cannot sleep, remain in bed and rest with an open torso rather than sitting up.

At 6 AM take another teaspoon of ColoZone with lemon juice and another at 8 AM. Drink warm water throughout. Omit the 8 AM dose if there have already been many bowels movements. Prepare your ama-reducing broth and kichuri when you get hungry.

When the bowel empties you will see aggregations of light green material and some unformed chaff floating on the water. Roughly count and notice size, shape and texture. Some people take photos for their brag book, I kid you not! Some of my ayurveda colleagues have had great success with this liver cleanse, done three times in 6-8 weeks, for their clients with myriad disorders. Western internists deny that the liver can be cleansed like this. Because we are asking the body to deal with a large amount of oil, make sure you are well enough to undertake this. The last thing some people need is the burden of all that oil.

As with every cleanse, allow a full day for rest and go to bed early the next night.

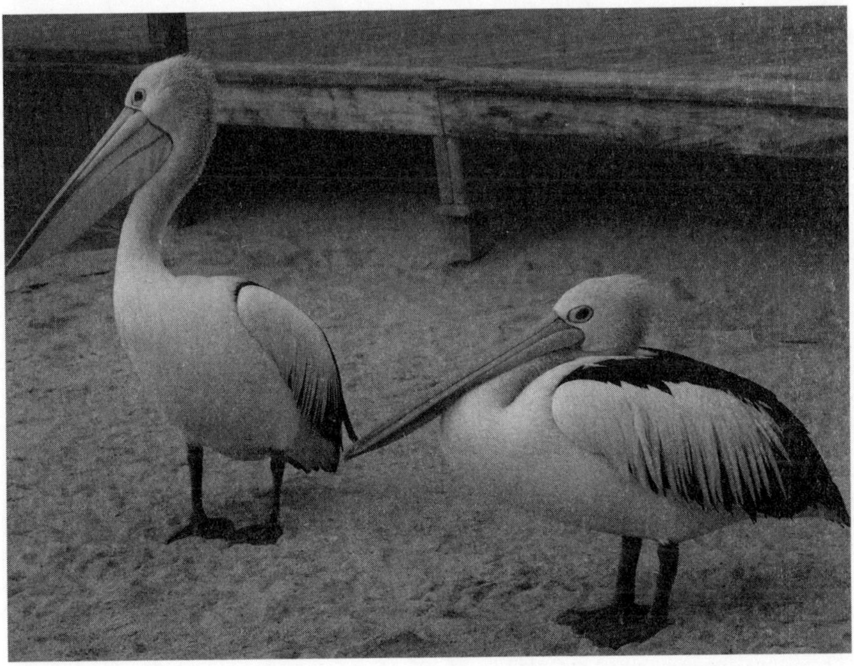

# NATURAL IMMUNITY

We are born with intrinsic immunity, a small amount that endures and can sustain the infant to the stage of receiving immunity from mother's milk; but it is not sufficient to sustain us as we grow. Acquired immunity is a result of the interaction with our new environment and proper digestion of all that we take in.

Our digestive system produces an assimible, nutrient-rich liquid that builds and nourishes our first body tissue, plasma. Refer to Part Two, THE SEVEN DHATU-S and MALA-S. All healthy tissues produce some ojas as a superior byproduct, with reproductive tissue producing the most. Ojas is considered a highly refined fluid-like substance that circulates throughout the body and imparts the glow and state of health, nourishing and connecting body, senses, mind and soul. Both AIDS and Chronic Fatigue are imbalances with low ojas. With high ojas we rarely become ill and if we do, we recover quickly. We are more stable and change is not a major challenge to the system.

Ojas is higher in males and in people that are more kapha-dominant. It is greatest in people neither very old nor very young, neither very tall nor very short, neither very fat nor very thin. It is decreased in people with excessive or scanty body hair, those who indulge in unhealthy food and is lower in cold, rainy and wintry weather.

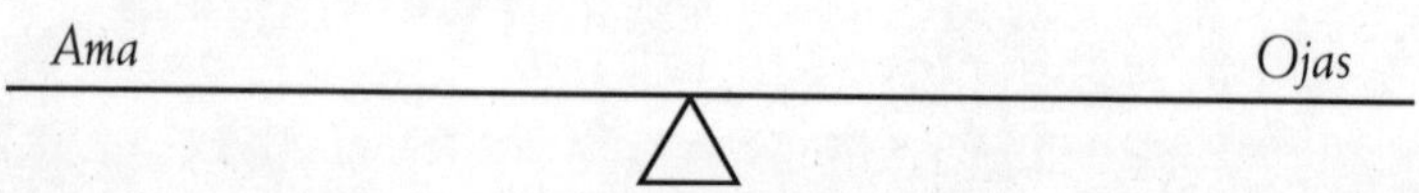


The less ama in the system the higher the natural immunity.

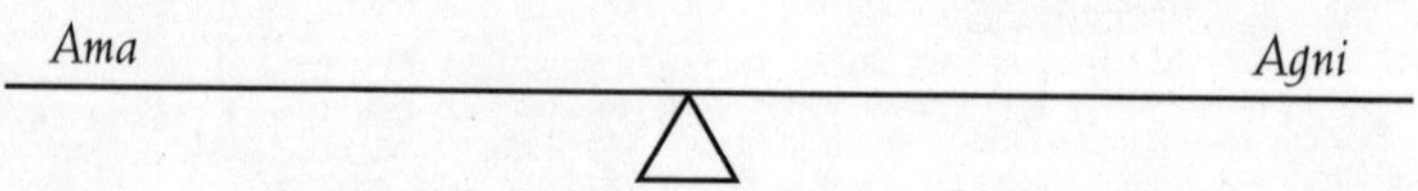


The more efficient a person's agni, the lower the ama. But if agni is too strong ama may increase. There are herbs that can raise and lower agni.

How can we enhance our natural immunity?

As always, diet and lifestyle are important pillars of pro-active support. Balancing agni and the dosha-s and removal of ama allows proper body functioning so that the diet and lifestyle can support our wellbeing. The internal and external environment we experience in our thoughts, feelings and the world around us also has an effect.

Sattwa in the person who cooks your food, in the food itself, while eating and in every aspect of life and relationships promotes ojas. Daily routine increases ojas. Foods that increase ojas are pure milk from contented cows, butter ghee, well-ripened fruit and fresh fruit juices, mung beans, fresh coconut in moderation, dates, grapes, figs, rice, sesame seeds and unfired honey. Proper use of the senses builds ojas. Devotion and selfless service do so as well.

Factors decreasing ojas are excessive physical activity, starving ourselves, intake of dry food and alcohol, excessive mentation and worry. Insomnia, injury, infections, wasting diseases, loss of body tissues, ingestion of foods antagonistic to yourself, stress and overindulgence or misuse of the senses all decrease ojas.

Foods that are generally antagonistic to ojas include all animal products, hard cheese, heavy, oily foods, leftover foods, excessively sour, salty or pungent food, mushrooms, peanuts, garlic, onions, caffeinated drinks, alcohol, tobacco and drugs.

There are ayurvedic preparations called rasayana-s that promote ojas. They are blends of tonic herbs, metals, fruits, gums, etc. and have specific methods of production which include the time of gathering, how it is cooked and specific blessings. They are a class of "leftovers" that have extreme positive benefit. High quality Chyawanprash is one of them.

Community is a source of ojas. The people we interact with can be supportive to our wellbeing. Make sure those around you are contributing to your ojas and you will be contributing to theirs.

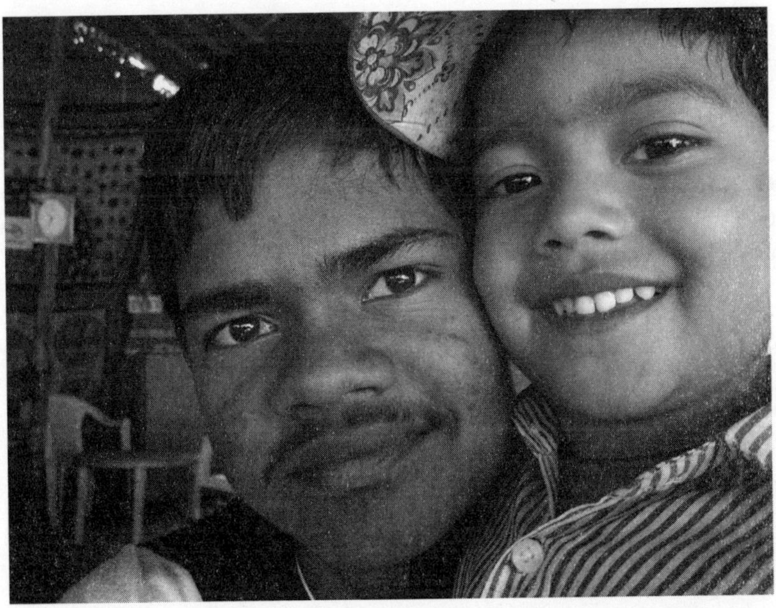

# THE PATHWAYS TO BALANCE

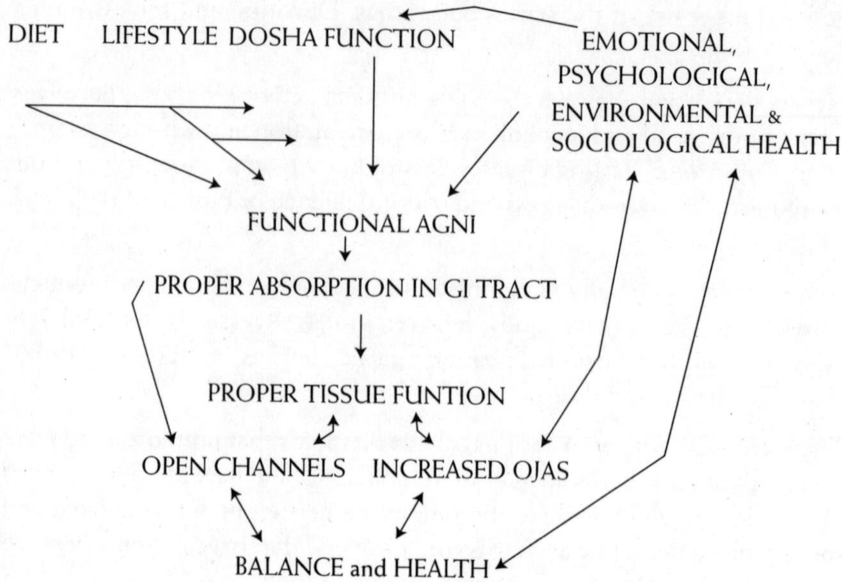


Signs and symptoms of balanced digestion (agni) include glowing complexion, bright eyes, strong digestion without constipation or diarrhea, ability to eat all foods, clear, straw-colored urine, normal, soft feces without a strong odor and maintenance of appropriate body weight for body type.

Ojas enhances nourishment, brings contentment, satisfaction, physical and mental endurance, resistance to disease, overall health and wellbeing and extends longevity. It is our vital reserve.

## THE PATHWAYS TO IMBALANCE

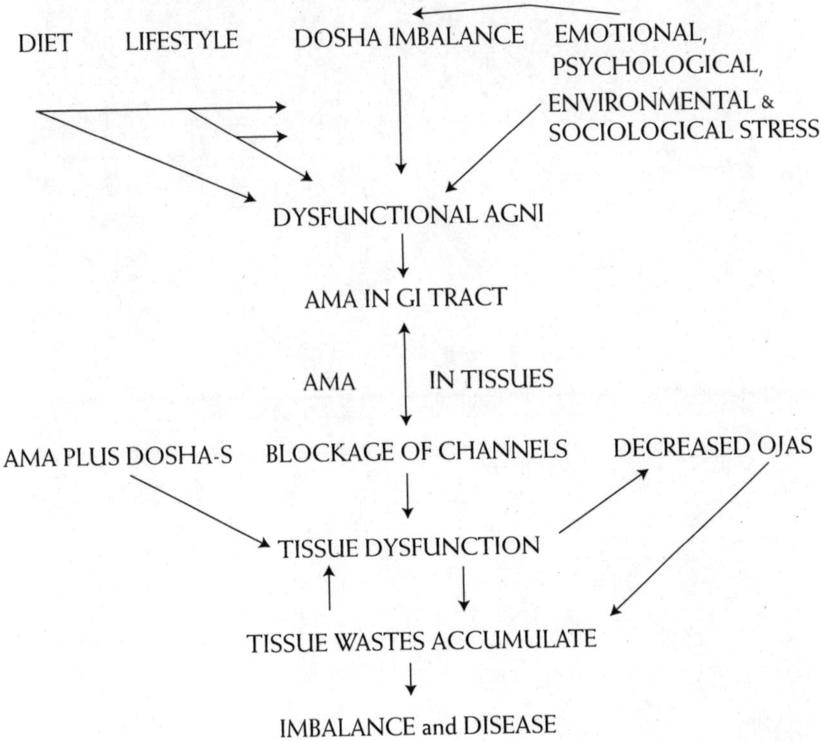


Signs and symptoms of ama include a furry coating on the tongue, drowsiness after meals, tiredness after minimal exertion, weight gain, joint pain and muscle aches, constipation or sticky stool, poor appetite, tiredness upon waking in the morning, frequent colds and influenza, bad breath, failing memory, low back pain not caused by injury, poor concentration, depression, mood changes, *Candida* infections and acne or boils.

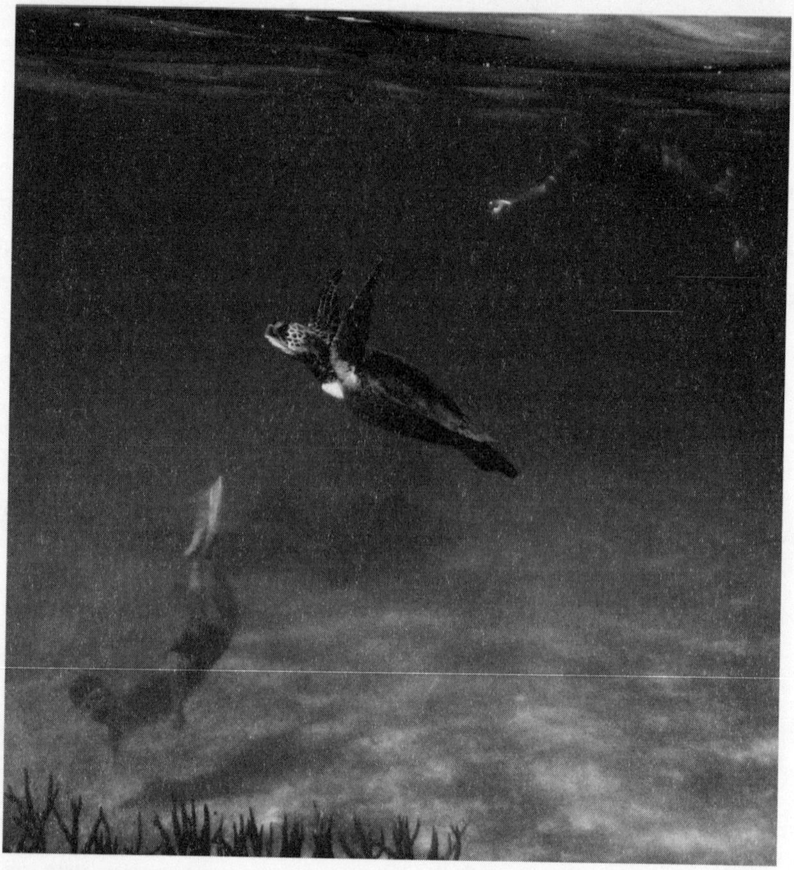

Methods and ingredients for wellness are right at our fingertips and always have been. When we are working with ayurvedic recommendations our innate wisdom is steadily revealed to us. That is what is meant to happen. Then we don't have to refer to a manual to know if we're feeling well and doing well.

As we remove ama and align with natural principles we find that we wish to continue the process. Our relationship to life has grown better. We feel clearer, more content, more altruistic, and more holistic. That is what is meant to happen. Then our energy flows freely and is available to use as we choose rather than being locked into distorted patterns.

The recommendations are so simple that at times they are ignored or we choose one and think the others are inconsequential. While one may be of help, more will provide for the best outcome.

May you accumulate ayurvedic health, your wealth.

May you enjoy the way.

## SHANTI NAMASKAR

SALUTE TO INNER PEACE

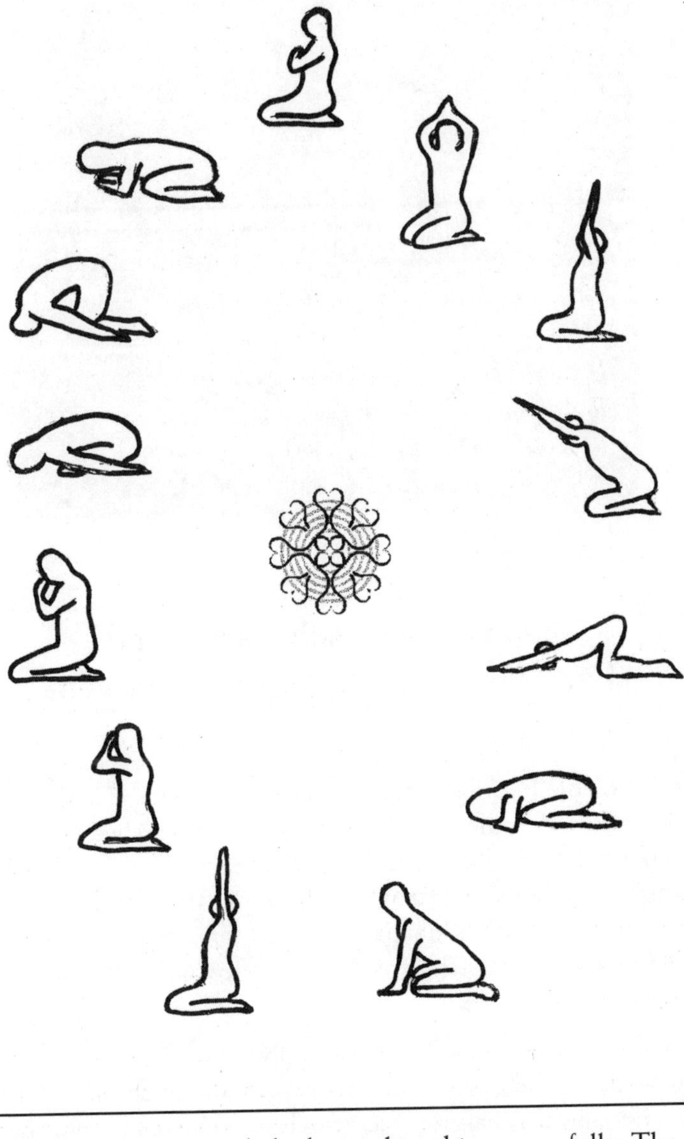

Begin at the top and proceed clockwise, breathing peacefully. The second posture is a twist, spiraled to both sides.

# PART FOUR

## Suggested Reading And Reference

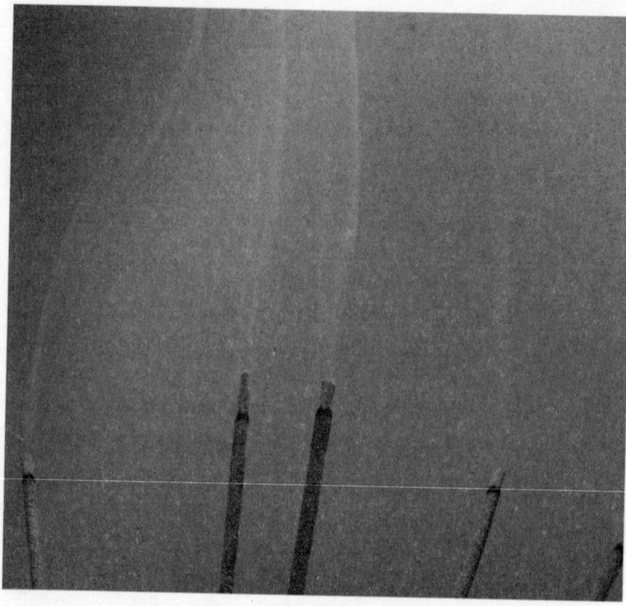

## Keraleeya Panchakarma and The Uniqueness of Kerala Ayurveda

Panchakarma means the fivefold treatment modalities. Pancha=five and karma=treatment. The classical panchakarma has ceased to be in practice in present times. A rather simplified form of it flourished in Kerala with their unique methods. The classical style speaks mainly of samshodhana (purifactory) methods to attain health, while the Kerala Panchakarma therapy consists of samshodhana as well as samshamana (palliative), i.e. it simultaneously expels the toxins and helps our body cure itself by strengthening it.

In fact the Keraleeya panchakarma is mainly pointed towards brumhanam, meaning body nourishment. The procedures are much more than five in number. The name panchakarma is used only in the symbolic sense here. Most of the panchakarma procedures in Kerala include both snehana (oleation) as well as swedana (sudation) done at the same time.

Shirodhara, Kayaseka, Pinda sweda, Anna lepa and Shirolepanam are the main procedures followed in Keraleeya panchakarma. Other treatments in classical method are also integrated like sneha basti, kashaya basti, udwarthanam, nasyam, tarpanam, patra potala swedam, choorna panda swedam; local bastis like janu, greeva and kati, pichu.

In Shirodhara, liquid media like medicated oils, milk, ghee, takra (buttermilk), decoction, etc. are placed in a dhara pot hung at an appropriate height and allowed to trickle slowly on the forehead. It is highly useful in patients suffering from diseases of head, and diseases like psychosis, epilepsy, neurosis, insomnia, etc.

When the same dhara is done for the whole body using cotton dipped in oil, it is called Kayaseka. This special treatment is of maximum popularity in Kerala. It provides simultaneous snehana (oleation) and swedana (sudation). In local language it is called pizichil. It is highly recommended for vata disorders.

Pinda sweda or njavara kizhi is the most popular Kerala panchakarma procedure. A bolus made in a cotton cloth with medicinal rice cooked in medicated milk is used to do massage. It is good for neuromuscular disorders, skin ailments and a good nourishment therapy. Similarly, when we smear the milk-cooked rice on the body it is called Annalepa. It is also a special Keralan treatment.

The smearing medicaments of cold potency on the head are called shirolepa. They are used in ailments of the head and neck, especially in cases of mental and brain disorders.

Many of the formulations used in Kerala are not seen in any of the three pillars of Ayurveda material medica – Charaka, Susruta and Vagbata. Also many treatment modalities which were given due importance developed to their peak level and evolved into a specific branch like that of Keraleeya panchakarma. An Ayurvedic materia medica used in Kerala by the name 'Sahasrayoga' (thousand medicinal preparations) refers to different preparations which were absent in any of the ancient scriptures. A wide array of medicines used in Ayurvedic practice evolved from Kerala. The treatments like Njavara kizhi, pizichil, talam, tala potichil, etc. are regarded as Kerala style by the scholars of Ayurveda.

**Compiled by Dr Subhash and Dr Visakh**

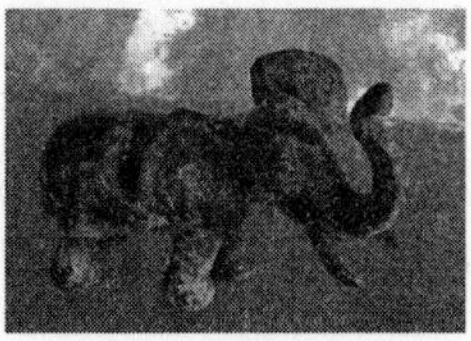

**Ayurdara**
**Vypeen Island**
**Kochi**
**Kerala, India**

# Reading and Websites

**A Woman's Best Medicine**
Lonsdorf, N, Butler, V, Brown, M. Penguin Putnam Inc., New York, 1995.

**Ageless Body, Timeless Mind**
Chopra, Dr Deepak. Three Rivers Press, New York, 1993.

**Ayurveda**
Ninivaggi, Dr Frank John. Praeger, Westport, CONN, 2008.

**Ayurveda, A Life in Balance**
Tiwari, Maya. Healing Arts Press, Rochester, VT, 1995.

**Ayurveda and Aromatherapy**
Miller, L and Miller, B. Lotus Press, Twin Lakes, WI, 1995.

**Ayurveda and Panchakarma**
Joshi, Dr Sunil V. Lotus Press, Twin Lakes, WI, 1996.

**Ayurveda and the Mind**
Frawley, Dr David. Lotus Press, Twin Lakes, WI, 1996.

**Ayurveda for Life**
Verma, Dr Vinod. Samuel Weiser Inc. York Beach, ME, 1997.

**Ayurveda for Women**
Svoboda, Dr Robert. Healing Arts Press, Rochester, VT, 2000.

**Ayurveda Revolutionized**
Tarabilda, Edward F. Lotus Press, Twin Lakes, WI, 1997.

**Ayurveda, the Gentle Health System**
Rhyner, Hans H. Sterling Publishing Co., New York, 1994.

**AyurVeda: The Ancient Indian Healing Art**
Gerson, Dr Scott. Element, Dorset, England, 1997.

**Ayurveda: The Science of Self-Healing**
Lad, Dr Vasant D. Lotus Press, Twin Lakes, WI, 1984.

**Ayurvedic Beauty Care**
Sachs, Melanie. Lotus Press, Twin Lakes, WI, 1994.

**Ayurvedic Cookbook**
Morningstar, Amadea and Desai, Urmila. Lotus Press, Twin Lakes, WI, 1990.

**Ayurvedic Cooking for Westerners**
Morningstar, Amadea. Lotus Press, Twin Lakes, WI, 1995.

**Ayurvedic Cooking**
Patel, Ramesh. Samhita Productions, Kensington, MD, 2003.

**The Ayurvedic Encyclopedia**
Tirtha, Swami Sada Shiva. Ayurvedic Holistic Center Press, Baysville, NY, 1998.

**Ayurvedic Healing: A Comprehensive Guide**
Frawley, Dr David. Lotus Press, Twin Lakes, WI, 2000.

**Ayurvedic Healing for Women**
Atreya. Lotus Press, Twin Lakes, WI, 1999.

**Ayurvedic Massage**
Johari, Harish. Healing Arts Press, Rochester, VT, 1996.

**Ayurvedic Secrets of Healing**
Tiwari, Maya. Lotus Press, Twin Lakes, WI, 1995.

**The Ayurvedic Year**
Brown, Christina. MQ Publications, London, England, 2002.

**Breath, Mind, and Consciousness**
Johari, Harish. Destiny Books, Rochester, VT, 1989.

**The Book of Ayurveda**
Morrison, Judith H. Gaia Books, London, England, 2005.

**The Chopra Center Cookbook**
Chopra, Dr D, Simon, Dr D, Backer, Leanne.
John Wiley and Sons, Hoboken, NJ, 2002.

**The Chopra Center Herbal Handbook**
Chopra, Dr D and Simon, Dr D. Three Rivers Press, NY, NY, 2000.

**Dangerous Beauty**
Dingle, Dr Peter and Brown, Toni. Self-Published, Perth, Australia, 1999.

**Dhanwantari, A Complete Guide to the Ayurvedic Life**
Johari, Harish. Healing Arts Press, Rochester, VT, 1998.

**Great Vegetarian Dishes**
Kurma Dasa. The Bhaktivedanta Book Trust, Botany Bay, Australia, 1990.

**Healing Cuisine**
Johari, Harish. Healing Arts Press, Rochester, VT, 2000.

**Healing with the Herbs of Life**
Tierra, Leslie. Crossing Press, NY, NY, 2001.

**The Heart of Yoga**
TKV Desikachar. Inner Traditions International, Rochester, VT, 1995.

**Heaven's Banquet**
Hospodor, Miriam. Plume, Penguin Group, NY, NY, 2001.

**The Hidden Secret of Ayurveda**
Svoboda, Dr Robert. The Ayurvedic Press, Alburquerque, NM, 2002.

**In Search of Mind**
TKV Desikachar. Krishnamacharya Yoga Mandiram, Chennai, India, 2001.

**Iyengar Yoga for Motherhood**
Iyengar, Geeta S, Keller, R and Khattab, K.
Stirling Publishing Co. Inc., N.Y., N.Y., 2010.

**Lost Secrets of Ayurvedic Acupuncture**
Ros, Dr Frank. Lotus Press, Twin Lakes, WI, 1994.

**Major Herbs of Ayurveda**
Self-published pamphlet by Dabur Company, India.

**The Mirror of Yoga**
Freeman, Richard. Shambala, Boston, MA, 2010.

**Modern Ailments, Ancient Remedies**
Kerr, Gillian, and Bloomfield, Dr Yvonne.
Landsdowne Press, Sydney, Australia, 1999.

**Nathamuni's Yoga Rahasya**
TKV Desikachar, translator.
Krishnamacharya Yoga Mandiram, Chennai, India, 1998.

**Nutritional Medicine: Fact and Fiction**
Tabrizian, Dr Igor. NRS Publishing, Greenwood, Western Australia, 2005.

**Perfect Health**
Chopra, Dr Deepak. Three Rivers Press, NY, NY, 1991.

**Perfect Health for Kids**
Douillard, Dr John. North Atlantic Books, Berkeley, CA, 2004.

**Phytotherapy, 50 Vital Herbs**
Chevalier, Andrew. Amberwood Press, Guildford, England, 1998.

**Planetary Herbology**
Tierra, Michael. Lotus Press, Twin Lakes, WI, 1988.

**Practical Ayurveda**
Atreya. Samuel Weiser Inc, York Beach, ME, 1988.

**Prakriti, Your Ayurvedic Constitution**
Svoboda, Dr Robert. published by Lotus Press, Twin Lakes WI, 1998.

**Quantum Healing**
Chopra, Dr Deepak. Bantam, USA, 1989.

**The Roots of Ayurveda**
Wujastyk, Dominik. Penguin Books, London, England, 2003.

**Sattwa Café**
Doherty, Meta B. Lotus Press, Twin Lakes, WI, 2006.

**Secrets of Ayurveda**
Warrier, G, Verma, H, Sullivan, K. Dorling Kindersley Ltd, Great Britain, 2001.

**Sick Homes**
Dingle, Dr Peter and Brown, Toni. Self-published, Perth, Australia, 2003.

**Tao and Dharma**
Svoboda, Dr Robert and Lade, Arnie. Lotus Press, Twin Lakes, WI, 1995.

**Textbook of Ayurveda Fundamental Principles**
Lad, Dr Vasant D. The Ayurvedic Press, Alburquerque, NM, 2002.

**Women's Power to Heal**
Tiwari, Maya. Mother Om Media,
distributed by Lotus Press, Twin Lakes, WI, 2007.

**Yoga and Ayurveda**
Frawley, Dr David. Lotus Press, Twin Lakes, WI, 1999.

**Yoga Beneath the Surface**
Ramaswami, Srivatsa and Hurwitz, Dave.
Marlowe and Company, New York, 2006.

**Yoga for Your Type**
Frawley, Dr David and Kozak, Sandra S. Lotus Press, Twin Lakes WI, 2001.

**Yoga Mala**
Sri K. Pattabhi Jois, North Point Press, New York, New York, 2010.

**Yoga of Heart**
Whitwell, Mark. Lantern Books, NY, 2004.

**Yoga of Herbs, an Ayurvedic Guide**
Frawley, Dr David and Lad, Dr Vasant D. Lotus Press, Twin Lakes, WI, 1986.

**Yoga Synergy**
Borg-Olivier, Simon and Machliss, Bianca.
Self-published, Sydney, Australia, 2002.

# WEBSITES

## including books, DVDs, treatments, herbs, etc.

www.ayurdara.de

www.davidwhyte.com

www.drsvoboda.com

www.heartofyoga.com

www.kym.org

www.lakshmiayurveda.com.au

www.LifeSpa.com

www.vedanet.com

www.yogasynergy.com.au

www.yogaworkshop.com

www.youtube.com

- Ayurveda, Forever Wellbeing, Part One
- Ayurveda, Forever Wellbeing, Part Two
- Ayurveda, Forever Wellbeing, Part Three
- Ayurveda, Forever Well Being, Yoga Program A
- Ayurveda, Forever Well Being, Yoga Program B
- Ayurveda, Forever Well Being, Yoga Program C
- Ayurveda, Forever Well Being, Yoga Program D
- Ayurveda, Forever Well Being, Yoga Extra

All photographs by Paul, Zack and Meta Doherty and friends.

Quest Dog Comic by Nate Doherty

# A Treasury Of Experiences

I still have a full time job in the corporate world and yet there is no conflict in practicing something that is traditional. Ayurveda, an ancient health system for modern wellbeing — actually not only modern. Forever Wellbeing, I would say that.
**–Ling**

In just 2 months, taking shatavari helped me more than any medication for period pain.
**–Wendy**

When my husband's skin started to itch and cause grief I mixed a paste of neem and chandana and it cleared the athletes foot but a detox will be needed to rebalance.
**–Jacqui**

Studying ayurveda has led me deeper into my spiritual journey.
**–Harry**

It started with me drinking hot water at work. With a little encouragement, okay, maybe a lot of encouragement, many workmates started drinking hot water too.
**–Dee**

Discovering Ayurveda was a godsend for me. Setting up a clinic has been a dream come true as I feel very fortunate in being able to practice this most beautiful science and fulfilling my dharma.
**–Karin**

We use ayurveda in a general sense in our home, for our children and ourselves. While we haven't delved deep, a little goes a long way.
**–Adam**

I came to ayurveda after one year travelling in India. My husband and I returned home with Giardia and Hepatitis A and were sick with chronic fatigue for two years. In Australia the western doctors couldn't really do anything for us. Since we fell sick in India we thought Indian medicine might be more able to help, so we tried a few different Ayurvedic doctors and I have to say some of them were complete quacks!!! One doctor even made me more sick by using cleansing herbs and purgation much too strongly on my already weak body.

When I found the right doctor I felt better within weeks. Within 3 months I was completely healthy, I was no longer underweight and I had the energy to enjoy my life again. I still see the same doctor now, many years later, and my whole family has a check up with him once or twice a year because prevention is the best cure. Ayurveda works on every level, I am healthier and stronger, I eat better without trying because I am in tune with what is good for me. I am more aware of my emotional health and the true causes of my ailments. It slots in really well with the yoga and meditation I was doing for many years before Ayurveda completed the picture. It's a whole philosophy of living, it takes dedication and commitment but the benefits are life changing.

And as a practitioner: I am naturally very left brained, and ayurveda appealed to me as a complete health science. I studied and measured and timed and memorised fine details, until the reality of ayurveda really hit me. Robert Svoboda, one of my mentors, describes ayurveda as a "qualitative science, not a quantitive science". You could also say it's more of an art. Either way this really changed my focus. Now my understanding as a practitioner has shifted to describing treatments as more elemental. A true Ayurvedic Doctor would study for six year and treat thousands of patients before being qualified. I am so grateful for everything I have learned, but it really is just the tip of the iceberg. It's more than a job, it's my life's work!
**–Julia**

I became more aware of my body through studying ayurveda. It started when I found that taking the rejuvenative jam called Chyawanprash at night kept me zinging for more hours than I wanted.
**–Amanda**

Even though I am a medical doctor, I can use ayurveda in my practice. It gives me a more dimensional understanding of my patients, physically and mentally.
**–Theresa**

When I first encountered ayurveda I was eating very healthily (so I thought) with lots of cold salads, wholegrain crackers, protein, dried fruit, fresh apple and pears and wondering 'why oh why was I so bloated all the time?' I'd cut out all the 'crap' (chocolate and processed foods) and was feeling very low about not seeing any improvement. My first appointment taught me about balancing my diet with my body type. I was predominantly 'air', and all the food I was eating was predominantly 'air' as well - no wonder I was manifesting a lot of 'air' in my belly. As soon as I started consuming more earthy, grounding foods I noticed an immediate improvement. Talk

about empowering! Over the years, the layers of knowledge unfolded and I learned to listen to my body, and I also now know what to do to rebalance when I don't!
**–Brenda**

Doing self-massage with ayurvedic oils definitely benefits me greatly in many ways - fantastic for my dry skin, nurturing time to myself and very grounding and calming for the mind. I always feel fantastic afterwards!
**–Angela**

Ayurveda brings a nurturing element to life and it brings softness. I have become very conscious of what this body and mind really mean and also connect spiritually. Emotionally I am stronger.
**–Bibi**

I have always been connected to nature so finding and using ayurveda was like being with a long lost friend.
**–George**

I have only taken on the hot water and bowel purge and that has made a good enough difference.
**–Ronnie**

I cook kichuri in the morning and take it to work every day. My friend asked why I bother. It's because I feel so much better because of it.
**–Sue**

My father has rheumatoid arthritis, which is beyond cure, and the western drugs taken over the years have done untold damage. However I finally persuaded him to do the lemon, ginger and honey drink and it did wonders for him. He kept it going for a while but my mother is a non-believer so it has now gone by the way. He got a clean bill of health check recently excepting the joint deformity so that is another testament to ayurveda.
**–Jacqui**

I understand more of what makes me what I am and other people too.
**–Adriana**

Excess internal heat was my problem. When I stopped eating three tomatoes a day, the heat instantly reduced. I couldn't believe it so I ate one tomato. The feeling of heat rose up again.
**–Gabriel**

I was flying backward and forward for work and that was unsettling for my nervous system. Sesame oil massage would soothe the agitation — when you're too frenetic - back into line. If I did it a few days in a row I felt much more strengthened and had more vigor.
**–Matt**

I enjoy the simplicity, thanks and peace in eating simple food.
**–Annabelle**

Ghee. Love ghee. Increasing the use of it since my yoga teacher said it is great for nourishing the nervous system and I feel more and more nourished.
**–Narelle**

I am sensitive to outer energy and with my self-massage and meditation I feel intrepid going out wearing my soft armor.
**–Nathelle**

Ayurvedic medicine has helped me solve the riddles and mysteries of health, which can be very elusive in today's society. Ayurveda gives a simple, clear and easy to understand explanation of how anybody can achieve and maintain extraordinarily powerful physical, emotional, mental and spiritual health.
**–Jeremy**

Starting with ayurveda study at home has led me to India to experience many forms of treatments. Eventually I came to know the habits of my mind that were driving me relentlessly, even to experience the treatments. I feel I have gotten wiser as I have gotten older and can now relax. I don't have to prove anything to myself.
**–Gary**

I was on a quest, seeking some help with my menstrual and fertility problems. I'm finely built and I used to think I was very healthy eating lots of salads and raw fresh food and drinking lots of fruit juices but from an ayurvedic perspective that was the wrong thing. I should have been having more warm food, unctuous foods, grounding foods. Even the yoga I was doing was fast moving and it was very aggravating. I completely changed my diet, looked into my lifestyle and became a lot more grounded. I did conceive and now have a child.
**–Leah**

Ayurveda is part of my cultural heritage as is gratitude and service.
**–Gopal**

The bowel cleanse allows my body to re-set and understand what is going on: it breaks the habits.
**–Annabelle**

Because of abhyanga, I now know that the skin is a large sense organ.
**–Paul**

I have found Ayurvedic treatments including dietary and lifestyle advice to be profoundly healing. In particular when I suffered headaches and a great deal of stress, the dosha model explained that vata had become deranged from racing around too much and prolonged mental work. Oil massages, dietary changes and a more regular, restful pattern returned me to optimal wellness quickly and with greater wisdom. From my understanding of Ayurveda I apply the principles of sattvaguna wherever possible in my environment both externally and internally. I also apply the guna qualities in my work as a naturopath and yoga therapist to my prescriptions of food, asana, lifestyle, meditation and herbal remedies.
**–Chandrika**

Ayurveda has provided me with a solid framework on which to base and build my whole life. Daily routine, practices I need to do to stay in balance, that has been a gift to not only help others but first and foremost keep myself in balance and live a happy healthy life.
**–Nikki**

In the colder months when I'm trying to settle after dinner and before bed I find ayurvedic milk very soothing and warming. I combine equal amounts of best quality available milk and water in a saucepan, add 2-3 slivers of fresh ginger, 3 bruised cardamom pods, ½-teaspoon turmeric powder and a few threads of saffron. I bring it to boil, reduce by half, sweeten to taste and sip before bed.
**–Michelle**

I suffered for many years from dermatitis on the hands, and nothing that doctors prescribed would help (apart from creams which would temporarily suppress the symptoms). After eight weeks of taking Safi, along with following a cleansing diet, the dermatitis completely disappeared and has not returned. After five weeks of panchakarma treatments at an ayurvedic hospital in Coimbatore all itchiness in the skin had gone and my palette felt completely clean and clear.
**–Lynn**

When I finally allowed myself some natural fats and oils, I found I slept better and was softer to people around me.
**–Gerard**

I now know that as we get older our body systems change and it's not always best to eat the foods and do the things we did when we were younger. As Dr Svoboda talked about, we can either glide down the other side or plummet! I still enjoy eating and doing what I do!
**–Barbara**

I eat only freshly cooked food in my home nowadays. We get hungry, we make some food up, we eat it. Simple as that! And I enjoy shopping weekly for yummy fresh things and alternate and vary what I buy. Nothing stays too long on the shelves or in the fridge.
**–Debbie**

Raising children with these teachings has kept them healthier and that makes me happier because when people ask me how I am, it's how my children are that matters most.
**–Robbie**

Aloe liquid provides menstrual regularity for me.
**–Maggie**

I have refined my food choices and my lifestyle choices without feeling it was a discipline.
**–Tanya**

Tongue scraping in the morning removes the layer of "sleep".
**–Annabelle**

It took time but I stopped breathing through my mouth. I found that I lost some extra weight in that process. My ayurvedic consultant explained that mouth breathing lowers the digestive fire, so I wasn't burning food efficiently.
**–Laura**

The baby massage is so lovely.
**–Gemma**

Ayurvedic treatments are truly profound. When people are complete with their treatments they actually feel love for themselves. And that's it, that's the key. Ayurveda is about life and love and living and healing.
**–Bibi**

# Afterword

Hi everyone, your tour guide here, baby boomer and wanted-to-be flower child but I was too shy to really live it.

Although the basic concepts of Ayurveda and the Five Great Elements are still the same, there is no doubt that there are new combinations and new ways of using them. Did the ancients foresee communication media to the extent that it is unfolding? The worldwide communication networks allow us to know almost instantly what is really happening in places of war and peace. We can retrieve information and learn about the research and discovery in any field that interests us, be kept amused by the creativity of people and darlingness of animals and be up to date about the lifestyles of the rich and famous and about each other.

The ancients proposed this: that the nature of *what is*, call it a personal God or the impersonal Brahman, periodically influences the creation of a whoosh of matter and anti-matter which lasts for eons and is then sucked back into potentiality, as an ongoing cosmic rhythm. So there's plenty of time and plenty of scenarios that have been and will be. If the Divine created all this in order to know itself, we itself know that we are that miraculous speck of consciousness on the barn floor of some farm in a galaxy far away, looped back on itself. An occasion for a barn dance!

I read in "Be Here Now, Remember" by Ram Dass that a teacher is someone who wants you to know the why and wherefore, the particulars, the information, the technology, the celebration of the doing and the knowing, who positions your thinking in a certain direction. A guru is someone who lives in the sea of love without the confines of any concepts because as soon as something is limited by definition, by definition we exclude the rest.

**Enjoy what ayurveda has to offer as information in the sea of love.**

**Meta in Perth, Australia**

**June 2011**

# Index

# H



# I



# J



# K



# L



# M



# N



# O



# P



# R



# S

## T



## V



## W



## Y